DANCING LIVES

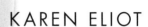

KAREN ELIOT

DANCING
LIVES

Five Female Dancers
from the Ballet d'Action
to Merce Cunningham

UNIVERSITY OF ILLINOIS PRESS
URBANA AND CHICAGO

© 2007 by Karen Eliot
All rights reserved
Manufactured in the United States of America
C 5 4 3 2 1
∞ This book is printed on acid-free paper.

Library of Congress Cataloging-in-Publication Data
Eliot, Karen, 1957–
Dancing lives : five female dancers from the
Ballet d'Action to Merce Cunningham / Karen Eliot.
p.   cm.
Includes bibliographical references and index.
ISBN-13 978-0-252-03250-9 (cloth : alk. paper)
ISBN-10 0-252-03250-0 (cloth : alk. paper)
1. Ballerinas—Biography. 2. Women dancers—Biography.
3. Ballet—History. 4. Modern dance—History.
I. Title.
GV1785.A1E55   2007
792.802'80922—dc22 [B]   2007011427

To my many inspired dance teachers,
especially Edith Vousden, Maggie Black,
Jocelyn Lorenz, Merce Cunningham,
and Chris Komar

CONTENTS

Illustrations follow page 90

ACKNOWLEDGMENTS

I FIRST ACKNOWLEDGE the women who are the subjects of this book, and note with sadness the passing of Moira Shearer, who died in 2006 while this book was in process. I am particularly grateful to my friend and former colleague Catherine Kerr, who graciously allowed me to interview her and document her story.

My work was supported by a Coca-Cola Grant for Research on Women and by the Department of Women's Studies at the Ohio State University. Additional generous support came from the Ohio State University College of the Arts, which awarded me several research grants to travel to archives and libraries in Europe and the United States. I am especially indebted to Beth Sullivan, former associate dean at Ohio State, for her initial encouragement of my project and for guiding me toward grant opportunities.

I am very grateful to my first readers, Jenny James Robinson and Hadassah Segal, who were nearly as excited and interested in the project as I was. I acknowledge with profound thanks Lynn Garafola's patient, thorough, and thought-provoking suggestions as she read various drafts of my manuscript. Her acute intelligence, lively intellectual curiosity, and rigorous scholarship are models for me. Her writing and her dedicated commitment to the field inspire me to persevere in dance history.

ACKNOWLEDGMENTS

Many thanks are due to the librarians and archivists who led me to valuable materials and often suggested avenues and resources I had not anticipated: the wonderful staff at the Bibliothèque de L'Opéra; Annette Fern, formerly of the Harvard Theatrical Collection; and the entire staff of the Jerome Robbins Dance Division at the New York Public Library for the Performing Arts, especially Patricia Rader, for materials on Baccelli, and Phil Karg, who helped me secure permissions for illustrations. I thank David Vaughan for allowing me to search through the archives at the Cunningham Dance Foundation and for his years of exemplary dance writing. Lise Friedman spent time talking with me and gave valuable advice on early drafts of the manuscript. Gino Bondi and Bettina Capello kindly and painstakingly made translations from eighteenth-century Italian newspapers. Jed Downhill has been enormously generous in allowing me to use his exquisite photographs of the Cunningham Dance Company. I thank Carol Bolton Betts at the University of Illinois Press for her meticulous editing and thoughtful suggestions.

Finally, I thank my family, who bore with me throughout.

DANCING LIVES

INTRODUCTION

EARLY IN THEIR LIVES, dancers learn the meaning of the word "work": it is the repetitious execution of demanding exercises in daily technique classes. It is what they do to improve their turns; lift their legs; rise to their toes; sustain a slow phrase of controlled motion in legs, back, and arms; flow through spirals and twists of the torso; leap from the floor and land with ease. Work is what they do to embody a choreographer's vision and what they must do on a nightly basis to achieve their fullest potential onstage. But when dancers pick up their dance bags and go home, they leave no record of what they have done. Though the physical changes accomplished through training and rehearsal are recorded in the bodies of individual dancers as they grow stronger, develop muscle tone, and train the neural pathways to accomplish a particularly challenging movement, the execution of the dancing that manifests this growth leaves no trace. The history of dancers' real work, then, is accessible only through secondary accounts. Rarely have the changes and developments in dance been examined through the lived bodies of the individuals who transform the art. No narrative of dance history can fully account for the critically important physical presence of the individual dancers whose work—both onstage and in daily classes and rehearsal studios—created the dance of their time; but the present book attempts to fill in gaps in our understanding of the changes in dance over time.

I start from the premise that dance history can be conceived as an embodied history. With that as my starting point, I explore a portion of dance history through a microscope rather than a telescope, bringing four European/Russian ballet dancers and an American modern dancer to the foreground and watching larger world events unfold as the backdrop to their experiences.

This is not a book for the dance specialist, who will find more detailed analyses of historical events and time periods in substantive works by Ivor Guest, Lynn Garafola, Sally Banes, David Vaughan, Marian Smith, John Chapman, and many others whose books and articles provided foundations upon which mine rests. Instead, I address an audience interested in dance history who have homes in other arts disciplines, as well as general students of dance history and people who are interested in the lives of working women across two hundred years of Western history. I have chosen to focus the lens of my microscope on five female dancers whose careers span the late eighteenth to the mid-twentieth centuries and who represent a cross section of training and performance in European and Russian ballet. Giovanna Baccelli (c. 1753–1801) was born in Venice, trained in Paris, and spent most of her working life in London; Adèle Dumilâtre (1821–1909) was born and trained in Paris and spent most of her working life at the Paris Opéra; Tamara Karsavina (1885–1978) was born and trained in St. Petersburg, performed with the Diaghilev Ballets Russes across Europe, branched out to perform on her own, and wrote, taught, and coached in England; and Moira Shearer (1926–2006) was born in Scotland, trained by British teachers in Rhodesia (now Zimbabwe) and by Russian and British teachers in London, performed with the International Ballet and the nascent Vic-Wells (later to become the Sadler's Wells Ballet), and then turned to an acting career in films and on stage. The American-born Catherine Kerr (1948–) began as a ballet dancer but found she was more attuned to the unconventional aesthetics of Merce Cunningham and went on to have a long and substantial career in the Merce Cunningham Dance Company.

These dancers passed down a legacy of French ballet technique, from the late eighteenth-century elegant *danse noble* and more sprightly *demi-caractère* styles that Giovanna Baccelli perfected in her career, to the highlighting of female virtuosity and the newly prominent place of the ballerina in the Romantic ballets embodied by Adèle Dumilâtre. Tamara Karsavina's life story demonstrates the infusion of Italian virtuosity into the more limpid Russian style. During Moira Shearer's career, the developing British ballet underwent a sometimes uncomfortable assimilation of teaching methods from all these classical traditions. Catherine Kerr began ballet classes as part of an overall plan of education and extracurricular activities that middle-class American families could provide for their young girls. Viewed as a group, these subjects demonstrate the changes in the education and class status of women in dance. Despite regional and temporal differences, all aspired to much the same goal. They all began to train as young girls and worked for years to become dancers. Though they represent distinctly different economic and social backgrounds, they mastered their art, and their names are, to some extent, remembered today.

Though each woman was recognized in her own time, these dancers are not necessarily the most famous of their eras; nor, in some cases, has their full significance as professional dancers been fully realized in historical accounts. Baccelli was something of a superstar in the late eighteenth century, but her reputation today has been superseded by those of the stunning male dancers who became known as the "gods of the dance," Gaetan and Auguste Vestris, and by the famous choreographer and dance theoretician Jean-Georges Noverre. All three were men with whom Baccelli's dance life would intersect. Yet, while their influence on the dance of their day is recognized, Baccelli's impact is not. Similarly overlooked is Adèle Dumilâtre, a nineteenth-century ballerina. During the height of the French Romantic ballet, Dumilâtre was what Alphonse Royer called a reputable second-tier ballerina.[1] Her name is today overshadowed by those of legendary (and, not coincidentally, non-French) ballerinas: Marie Taglioni, Fanny Elssler, Fanny Cerrito, Carlotta Grisi, and Lucille Grahn. Tamara Karsavina, a nearly legendary ballerina with the Diaghilev Ballets Russes during the early years of the twentieth century, is well known as the most significant interpreter of Michel Fokine's ballets and the partner of Vaslav Nijinsky. Less well known is that Karsavina also had a substantial professional career outside of her work with the Ballets Russes. Her influence as a teacher, writer, and performer beyond her work with Diaghilev, and her substantial impact on the British ballet, is frequently eclipsed by the stories of the nearly mythic contemporary ballerina, Anna Pavlova, who toured widely. Although Moira Shearer is beloved by many dance watchers and movie aficionados, her ballet career was notoriously obscured by that of the British prima ballerina Margot Fonteyn. Shearer was noted as a luminous young star during the 1940s and was one of a number of young talented ballerinas "to be watched," but her ballet career ended prematurely, possibly because she reached the glass ceiling that prohibited talented female dancers from attaining Fonteyn's level of stardom. And Kerr, though acknowledged by other company dancers as having had a substantial and very fruitful relationship with Merce Cunningham, is little known outside the circles of intimate Cunningham followers.

Dancers are the stuff of which dance history is made, but there are few histories focusing on their lives as working professionals. While readers may have access to biographies of ballet superstars, they rarely encounter a history charted through the working lives of female dancers. Amy Koritz, for one, has addressed the omission of the performer's side of the story in dance history. "Despite a concerted effort in the last two decades to expand and multiply our narratives of cultural history," she writes, "we are still likely to assume that those artists whose voices are most heard and accomplishments frequently cited are simply the most deserving of that attention." Koritz notes Walter Benjamin's reminder that "our 'documents of civilization' are tainted by the barbarism that erased those unheard voices."[2]

One problem for the dance historian is, as Benjamin might have put it, the "erasure" of dancers' experiences. Dance is hard to capture in words, and the difficulty of a historical project documenting dancers' careers is magnified when the historian sets about to map out the physical, emotional, and kinesthetic experiences of dancers dancing. In part, the dancer as artist and working woman has been deemed unworthy of serious scholarship for this very reason: her work is ephemeral and blatantly nonliterate. Like most other working men and women, dancers do not generally perceive their lives as "history in the making." With occasional exceptions, they do not record the everyday occurrences of their lives as these are experienced as a series of ongoing tasks, quotidian duties along with personal defeats and joys.[3] Under the best of circumstances, the history of dance is severely underdocumented, in part because dance is popularly considered a woman's "diversion." Koritz believes that the marginalization of dance studies has resulted partly from the association of dance with "femininity" and "female erotic display." Over time, however, as dance became a more widely recognized and less culturally degraded form, women performers were regarded as empty vessels to be filled. The "artist" whose work was worthy of scholarship, and who might secure a place in the halls of academe, was assumed to be the male "author," the choreographer or director of the work. Scholars and critics of Western art have tended to focus primary attention on the so-called creator of the work at the expense of the performer, or in other words, to concentrate on the implicit (male) author of the work at the expense of what is assumed to be its (female) interpreter.[4] In reality, however, such a distinction in performative and creative roles is nowhere less clear than in the realm of dance, where there are fluid boundaries between the choreographer and the artist whose daily work involves bringing to life the choreographer's vision. In fact, the separation between the "ideas" of the work's choreographer and the neural impulses and kinetic potential of the dancer's body may even change with each performance of the work.

I have chosen to concentrate on the participation of five female dancers, but it goes without saying that men too are and have been dancers, just as women are and have been choreographers. However, while the presence of male dancers has varied widely over time, women have rarely been absent as performers on the stage. Women have been dancing for centuries and there is no question that dance is a profession that is popularly associated with women. Sally Banes explains that, "like so many women involved in dance, I long felt that an explicit feminist analysis was simply unnecessary in a highly feminized field, where many of the leading figures—both artists and scholars—are women." But, after further reflection, Banes concluded that "the discipline of dance history has only very recently begun to be examined from a feminist perspective, and there are very few models."[5]

The present book is an effort to help fill that gap: to see the history of the times as lived by individual female dancers. The focus is on the working dancers whose careers, in important ways, represent the major issues in the dance of their times. In each chapter I discuss the individual dancer's social and economic status; her education and dance training; the cultural expectations about dance in her time; and her route to a professional career. I frame each woman within her own cultural world by examining specific works in which she danced, and by analyzing the significant debates of the day about choreography and dance. I am also concerned, however, with their individual lives as women—as wives, daughters, sisters, mothers, students—and these issues play into the stories of their lives as well.

The difficulty of recording changes marked through the daily work of dancers' bodies, as well as the overall nonliteracy of the field, presents the dance historian with a number of challenges. In spite of the public and theatrical aspects of these women's careers, there is little to document their working lives and kinesthetic experiences as dancers. I found myself using unconventional historical tools, drawing my hypotheses from such sources as paintings and sculptures, novels, poems, and commercial films. In the introduction to the fourth volume of the series entitled A History of Private Life, Michelle Perrot frames the dilemma this way: "We have been forced to cobble together a narrative from fragmentary findings."[6] In my effort to delve into the more private—less easily articulated—aspects of a dancer's experience, I find that I too have "cobbled" together my narratives; nevertheless, in each instance, I have constructed an individual dancer's world based on the best available resources, suggesting possible responses or motivations when concrete data is not to be found. In a sense, I have pursued what Toni Morrison calls "literary archeology." According to Morrison, writing a novel based on historical events requires an intuitive understanding of the past, for such a process requires that "on the basis of some information and a little bit of guesswork you journey to a site to see what remains were left behind and to reconstruct the world that these remains imply."[7] Amanda Foreman, a biographer, describes her more orthodox historical process in much the same way: "Finally, it is intuition and a sympathy with the past which supply the last missing pieces." I perceive my task in similar fashion: while seeking information, I simultaneously engage in "creative empathy" to fit together the pieces of the women's experiences.[8] Empathy guides the process of writing about dancers' lives, but my reconstruction of their careers and their experiences in dance is based on the preserved shards of dance history.

John Lewis Gaddis, in his book *The Landscape of History: How Historians Map the Past*, describes the historian's process as one of making choices about how to represent the past, how to describe the territory and choose the features to highlight. A mapmaker, says Gaddis, goes through a related decision-making process in selecting a mode of representation: "Maps vary scale and content according to need. A world map has a different purpose from one intended to identify bicycle paths or garbage dumps. Nor are maps free from preconceptions. There's always some prior reason for what's shown and not shown."[9] This book redraws the landscape of dance history; it creates a map highlighting the lives of five female dancers who embodied the dance of their times. It represents dance history as it has been created on, in, and through their bodies.

1

GIOVANNA
BACCELLI

HER INVITING SMILE, lustrous eyes, dark hair, and slender, oval face draw a cluster of viewers who gather in front of her full-length portrait. Thomas Gainsborough's painting of the ballerina Giovanna Baccelli, shown in her role in the ballet *Les amans surpris,* makes museum-goers pause; unlike more stately eighteenth-century portraits, this one captures motion: the dancer's movement in space. Viewers are drawn to Baccelli's physical beauty and respond kinesthetically to her dancing. Gainsborough's full-length portrait of Baccelli, first exhibited at London's Royal Academy of Art in 1782, is now housed in Tate Britain.[1] As I contemplated what is described as "one of the most sparkling and lively full-lengths of [Gainsborough's] mature period,"[2] I could only speculate about the inevitable years of discipline and training, the rough edges omitted in this portrait of insouciant ease and grace.

Giovanna Baccelli was an alluring female subject for artists of the late eighteenth century. Her lively features, her poise in movement, and her soft but vivacious femininity intrigued them. Artists including Thomas Gainsborough, Joshua Reynolds, John Boydell, and John Baptiste Locatelli have left portraits, lithographs, drawings, and sculptures as testimony to her many attractions. Yet the Venetian-born Baccelli was also a notable ballerina who, in the male-dominated world of eighteenth-century ballet, partnered significant male superstars, including the Vestris father and son, and appeared in choreography by noted ballet masters such as Jean-Georges Noverre, Louis Simonet, Dominique Lefèvre, and Francesco Clerico. I wonder, though, if Baccelli would be remembered today—alongside her better-known male dance colleagues—had she not also been a beautiful and engaging model for painters and sculptors.

Elizabeth Einberg, an art historian, links Gainsborough's portrait to a time, late in his life, when the painter engaged in novel efforts to capture movement and the effects of light and space. The Baccelli portrait allowed Gainsborough to experiment with a number of new approaches to depicting a figure in landscape; the result, says Einberg, was a "uniquely harmonious combination of painter, sitter and technique." The painter captures Baccelli in mid-movement, her slender foot extended in its heeled slipper. While the movement is ongoing, the portrait also evokes a sense of overall balance and equilibrium. The ballerina shows a trained vertical aplomb—a sense of poise and ease—through her spine, ribcage, neck, and head; her left arm is extended so that she holds the edge of her skirt at just the angle to balance the line of her arched and outwardly rotated foot. There is volume and dimension in the movement of the trees, in the skies and foothills in the background, in the curving of the dancer's arm, the beribboned sleeve tucked behind her back, and in the inclination of her head and the draping of her skirt. Baccelli appears capable of choosing at any moment to bend her well-turned-out knee in a *plié* and to step out to balance on the ball of her extended right foot. Of the possible qualities Gainsborough might have selected, it was her physical beauty and serene control that captured the painter's imagination.

Deliberately flouting eighteenth-century conventions of genre-painting and portraiture, Gainsborough sought to depict the woman as dancer. Sir Joshua Reynolds, on the other hand, was intrigued by the ballerina as courtesan.[3] While it was probably Baccelli's idea that she be painted by Gainsborough, it was at the behest of her then lover, John Frederick Sackville, third Duke of Dorset, that Reynolds created his portrait of the ballerina. In his 1783 commission Reynolds chose to subject La Baccelli "to an elaborate programme of Venetian colouring and allusions to Dionysiac revels . . . and the stage."[4] The Reynolds portrait, an engraving of which was made by J. R. Smith in 1783, depicts Baccelli in her theatrical garb as a Bacchante. Baccelli is clearly a woman of the theater; warm from her efforts on the stage, she emerges to public view in a seductive state of dishevelment. She appears to step out from a dark and lush forest, a theatrical backdrop that hints at untamed wildness and the promise of revelry. The ballerina has just removed her mask, and she glances at her viewer over her bare right shoulder. A lock of hair curls over the right side of her back, and garlands of vines and leaves adorn her head. Her dark, melting eyes look at the viewer: her glance is direct, unaffected, even gentle.

———

Details about Baccelli's early years—prior to her arrival in England, her performing seasons in London, and her residence at Knole as the duke's mistress—are fragmentary. She was born in Venice, circa 1753, to an itinerant Italian theater family. Her family name was Zanerini, and her sister, "Argentine" Zanerini, was a popular actress at the Comédie-Italienne.[5] It may be that Baccelli's mother, Antonietta Rosa Baccelli, remarried and that Giovanna (sometimes called Gianetta, or Janetta) was the daughter of the second husband.[6] Apparently Giovanna was fluent in French and Italian and she could also speak and write in English.[7] Her first London appearance occurred in November 1774 when she danced as the Rose in *Le ballet des fleurs,* a *divertissement* from Rameau's opera *Les Indes galantes.*[8]

Although not much is known about the Zanerini and Baccelli families, something of their peripatetic existence can be inferred through descriptions of numerous other theatrical clans who traveled throughout the fairgrounds and courts of Europe for hundreds of years. Descendants of these long-established families frequently included skilled fairground entertainers, teachers, acrobats, dancing masters, and classically trained dancers whose careers established them in the great opera houses. Marian Hannah Winter reports on one such dynasty, the Chiarinis, whose members included a family of noted rope dancers. Numbered among the wandering Chiarini clan were also at least one equestrienne, a dancing master and a *premier danseur* at La Scala, tight-rope performers, and a branch of the family that ran a school of mime in Vienna for circus children.[9]

Even the renowned Vestris family had nomadic origins. Born in Florence, Gaétan Vestris established himself as preeminent at the Paris Opéra. Earlier, however, according to the dance historian Ivor Guest, when the family first arrived in Paris in 1747, "an aura of adventure and glamour, louchely spiced though it was, surrounded these colourful immigrants." Rambling through Europe, the family survived on the musical and dance talents of the children.[10] In times of penury, Guest notes, it was particularly useful that "the girls were so precociously attractive, for in the course of their wanderings through Italy and into Austria, Gaétan and his brother Angiolo were here and there able to pick up engagements, while their mother and the eldest girls blatantly capitalised on their sexual charms."[11] Similarly, there would be little question that throughout her career Baccelli would call upon her plentiful reserves of "sexual charms" to support herself, though evidence suggests she remained faithful to the duke for many years.

Two of the male superstars of the Vestris clan, Gaétan and his son Auguste, were to cross Baccelli's career path, and Auguste would later become one of her most important dancing partners. Like the Vestris men and many of the other significant dancers of the day, Baccelli was trained in Paris. She then launched her career at King's Theatre, the opera house in London's Haymarket, where she danced from 1774 to 1783, often paired with Auguste. Once she was more firmly established in her career, she also performed selected seasons at the Paris Opéra (her debut there as guest ballerina occurred in 1782), and she returned to her native Venice on numerous occasions, performing at the Teatro San Benedetto, particularly during the Carnevale and Festival of Ascension ceremonies, until at least 1789.

By 1779, Baccelli—an effervescent woman—had been acknowledged as the mistress of the third Duke of Dorset and had moved with him to his family estate. Vita Sackville-West, in *Knole and the Sackvilles,* her anecdotal account of her ancestral home, describes the duke as having (at least for a time) "lost his head completely over her"; he caused a scandal in the neighborhood when he took Baccelli to a ball in Sevenoaks and decked her out in the family jewels.[12] Baccelli's status as a well-known ballerina and, perhaps more important, her acknowledged role as courtesan gave her public notoriety in what the art historian Mark Hallet has called the late eighteenth-century's "recognisably modern economy of celebrity."[13]

John Fredrick Sackville and his ballerina kept up a steady round of social activities during their years together. He was a worldly man, renowned as much for his notorious liaisons as for his extensive art collection.[14] In 1769, when he was twenty-four, John Frederick Sackville succeeded his uncle to become the third Duke of Dorset and then took over the extensive lands at Knole. The following year, he embarked on the Grand Tour of Italy, visiting collections and buying artworks in Rome, Naples, Florence, and Venice. The duke was also an avid cricket player and managed to make his little town of Sevenoaks a center for the sport.[15] Robert Sackville-West writes that although Dorset was not successful in introducing previous mistresses to the game, Baccelli did become interested. In a touching gesture of maternal affection, she purchased a cricket bat and stumps for her one surviving son by the duke, the younger John Frederick, born probably in 1779.[16]

Although the ballerina's domestic existence at the duke's rambling estate may have insulated her from public attention, rural retreat effectively opened her life to gossipy speculation. The widely circulated newspapers of the day gave "ever-more detailed accounts, both fawning and acidic, of the lives and activities of the men and women they considered to be of public interest," and Baccelli was not immune to examination.[17] A glancing reference in the *Morning Herald* of January, 3, 1783, underlined the degree to which public curiosity was aroused by the duke and his mistress: "Baccelli's return occasioned her amorous partner to take several steps to convince her of his extreme attention; with this view he met her immediately after she landed in England and conducted her to his seat!"

There is no way to determine Baccelli's relationships with her dance colleagues, yet press reports fueled speculation about Baccelli's professional rivals. The *Morning Herald* for September 27, 1781, suggested that Baccelli was put out at the terms offered her rival, Mademoiselle Théodore: "One of the *Operatical cognoscenti* informs us, that Madame Théodore has at length obtained her terms of the Managers for her light footed performances the approaching season; in consequence of which, the Baccelli retires in high dudgeon, but it is to be hoped, only *pro tempere!*"

Competing interests may have contributed to the unfavorable reviews of Baccelli's performances that occasionally surfaced.[18] The *Morning Herald and Daily Advertiser* of March 31, 1783, announced Baccelli's forthcoming *pas de deux,* with Mademoiselle Rossi wearing men's costume, in Charles Lepicq's new ballet, *Alexander and Roxanna.* The disparaging reviewer remarked that Baccelli "must feel bold indeed . . . to encounter such a rival as Mademoiselle Rossi, who besides her acknowledged merit, has this advantage, that having practised the whole season, she must be far more *en train* than the former, whose limbs must be stiffened with the chill of idleness, she having spent the whole of her time since her return from Paris in a kind of *otium cum dignate.*"[19]

Highfill, Burnim, and Langhans have suggested that Baccelli was less than perfectly attentive to her career, commenting that "Mlle Baccelli's relationship with the Duke seems to have prevented a full-time commitment to her profession, and in some years she did not come on until mid-season or later."[20] While the review from the *Morning Herald* undoubtedly alluded to Baccelli's illicit relationship with the duke, reviews were sometimes planted by partisans, and the popular press could be tapped to spread salacious gossip. Further, then as now, dancers were occasionally forced to postpone or cancel appearances due to injuries and illnesses, and bad press could result, though these circumstances were commonly reported in advance in the newspapers.[21]

The duke, who was appointed ambassador to the court of Louis XVI in 1783, probably did not ever compel Baccelli to neglect her career, and he may have even interceded on her behalf so that she could dance as a guest ballerina at the Paris Opéra during the 1782 season. Ivor Guest suggests, however, that her relationship with Dorset may have led her to give up dance when she "retired" during the 1784–85 season. But her time away from the stage was short-lived. She was subsequently re-engaged in London, though she was contracted for only a short period, which suggests she was experiencing another pressure. Once again her probable personal concerns were reported in the press, where it was speculated that another Opéra dancer, a Mademoiselle Gervais, had taken her place in the duke's bed.[22]

In any event, the British press kept track of Baccelli's affairs. The report from the *Morning Herald and Daily Advertiser* on February 9, 1785, was that "Madame Baccelli lives in great splendour in Paris, and no lady more truly deserves good fortune than herself. Her house is the resort of all the fashionable English in that gay metropolis and it is the chief pleasure and study of her life to shew her gratitude to our nation for the protection with which she was honoured by our nobility." An article from the *Morning Herald* on January 27, 1786, eagerly anticipated her return to London, reporting that "Madam Baccelli will quit Paris towards the conclusion of next month, and certainly begin about the first week in March, if not earlier, to resume her department in the scene of graceful agility."

Three days later, however, Baccelli was reportedly sick. Was she "indisposed" as a result of Dorset's flirtations with other dancers? The same newspaper noted, "The report behind the Opera scenes on Saturday evening was that Baccelli had been seized with an apoplectic stroke, and lay dangerously ill at the Duke of Dorset's hotel in Paris. The echo of these unpleasing tidings reached the pit, where it met the belief of many." On February 4, 1786, again came news from the *Morning Herald* concerning Baccelli's illness: "Madame Baccelli has been indisposed, but not in so violent a degree as report stated a few days since; she will no doubt be in England in about a month."

When she returned at last to English audiences, she was warmly applauded. According to her fans, Baccelli's technique had improved during her time in Paris, as she had taken the opportunity to continue her studies with Pierre Gardel.[23] On April 3, 1786, the *Morning Herald* reported:

> The new divertissement, intituled *Cupid turned Gardner* [*sic*], performed on Saturday evening, is the composition of Mr. Degville, one of the balletmasters. It was evidently calculated to introduce Madame Baccelli.... The re-appearance of that excellent performer, after so long an absence from a stage where she always was, and deserved to be welcome, was the more acceptable to the lovers of graceful and animated dancing. That she is astonishingly improved, and by her example verifies the truth of the remark, of which the French are

so proud, tho' of a very light importance, that in point of dancing, the Paris School "can perfect perfection itself."

After 1789, when Dorset left his post as ambassador, Baccelli's picture begins to recede gradually from view and it is more difficult to track her professional career. Dorset, apparently deeply affected by the devastation and death he witnessed in revolutionary France, also fell victim to a familial "melancholia." He made clear his intention to forgo his youthful indiscretions and to rescue the family fortunes, apprising the Duchess of Devonshire, for one, that he planned to marry the first heiress who would have him.[24] According to Einberg, the "affectionate tone" in which Dorset wrote of Baccelli suggests that "her natural sweetness of temper and vivacity must have been a great antidote for gathering depression."[25] In any event, Dorset married Arabella Cope, who brought him a dowry of £140,000; Baccelli took an annual pension of £400 and left her son to be raised as a gentleman by the duke. When Arabella Cope arrived at Knole, many of the duke's art treasures—including the Gainsborough portrait and a provocative Locatelli sculpture depicting an elegant nude, prone Baccelli—were discreetly exiled to the basement.

On leaving Knole, Baccelli entered into a relationship with Henry Herbert, tenth Earl of Pembroke, a longtime friend. She remained with the earl until he died in 1794. In August 1792, after dining with Pembroke, James Boswell spoke harshly of Pembroke's infatuation with Baccelli: "I felt it strange, and regretted it, that so amiable a man should have contracted such dissolute habits, and at this very time, instead of living respectably with his charming Countess, had Baccelli, the superannuated dancing Courtesan, in a *Cassino* in the neighborhood."[26]

Given Boswell's dissolute habits and his own refusal to maintain a respectable lifestyle, his denigration of Pembroke's affair is puzzling. One can only speculate that it was Baccelli's aging body that made her a less than attractive mistress from Boswell's point of view. After Pembroke's death, Baccelli evidently married a Mr. James Carey, who, Elizabeth Einberg writes, "took good care of her affairs" until her death in 1801.[27] Meanwhile, Baccelli's son received the instruction befitting a young gentleman and later embarked on a military career, first as a lieutenant and later as a captain in the 69th Regiment of Foot. Between 1796 and 1798, the regiment was stationed in Santo Domingo, where young Sackville contracted "a deadly feaver" and died.[28] Prior to his death, however, he had fathered the child of a pastry cook's daughter. Although Baccelli frequently sent money to support her grandson, "she saw to it that the boy's mother should in no way benefit from her will."[29] Her son's association with the daughter of a common cook was clearly an embarrassment both to the Sackville family and to his mother, the ballerina.

━━━

Baccelli's status in ballet history is assured in part because of her interactions with important *danseurs* like Vestris *père* and *fils*, and with ballet masters such as Jean-Georges Noverre. Her professional career during the 1770s and 80s coincided with a tumultuous and revolutionary period in the history of western Europe, and a similarly energized period of experimentation in literature, theater, and the visual arts. The dance historian John Chapman describes one of the pivotal debates occurring in ballet: on the one hand, some dancers were exploring virtuosity and pushing their technical prowess, while another group advocated a more aristocratic dance style of grace, dignity, and the avoidance of tension and strain. "Though the controversy neared its most intense period in 1800," Chapman writes, "as early as 1760 Jean-Georges Noverre (1727–1810) was pleading, in his extremely influential *Lettres sur la danse*, that his fellow artists renounce *entrechats* and *cabrioles*, abandon *tours de force*, which he considered to be meaningless."[30]

Emerging as a dancer in the midst of this debate, Baccelli, like her frequent dance partner, the *dieu de la danse*, Auguste Vestris (1760–1842), would learn to assimilate the theatrical, expressive elements of dance advocated by Noverre, while also acquiring significant technical skills. Vestris overwhelmed "the dance world with his spectacularly athletic technique." His celebrity status and his powerful presence on European stages spurred other dancers to imitate his technical innovations. While most lacked his supreme expertise and refined ease in movement, many dancers attempted the multiple pirouettes and beats he tossed off with seeming abandon. In large part, the changing approaches to virtuosity were embodied in the dance styles of the Vestris father and son. Gaétan exemplified the older, more dignified *danse noble* style, while his son, Auguste, was a "brilliant exponent of the *demi-caractère*, a style that allowed him scope for technical innovation and pantomimic expression."[31] Gaétan Vestris (1729–1808) maintained the aristocratic order in his refined and polished demeanor; Auguste, on the other hand, innovated by collapsing the boundaries between the genres. More than simply creating a shift in emphasis, Chapman says, Auguste changed the face of the dance: he "render[ed] the noble dance obsolete. Previous innovations took place within the traditional system; Vestris changed the system."[32]

Evidence suggests that, like Auguste Vestris, Baccelli was a new dancer for a new era. Her dancing, like his, went through a transformation; her training and the course of her career indicate that her professional life mirrored that of Vestris *fils*. While the younger Vestris's accomplishments are more fully documented, Baccelli was similarly acclaimed for her refined elegance and her superlative execution of virtuoso feats. Baccelli and Vestris broke established boundaries in achieving extraordinarily demanding technical feats, while they also explored the dramatic demands of *ballets d'actions* created by Jean-Georges Noverre and other like-minded *maîtres*, who required dancers to communicate through mimed gesture and movement.[33] Throughout her career, Baccelli was noted for the elegance, grace, and refined ease characteristic of the *danse noble* genre. Meanwhile, an examination of her repertory suggests that she also assumed an array of challenging theatrical roles and learned, over time, to expand her dramatic range.

The technical demands of the eighteenth-century dance class have been recorded in the extensive writings of European dance masters. A survey of these writings lends insights into the work that commonly went on in the ballet studio. Eighteenth-century ballet dancers trained intensively and began their study in childhood for a profession that required long hours of dedicated and disciplined exercise. Their dance training encouraged principles of balance, proportion, and symmetry; and, the manuals suggest, one purpose of the dance class was to shape the body into legible but also pleasing and expressive postures.

Giovanni-Andrea Gallini, whose 1762 publication *A Treatise on the Art of Dancing* went into three editions, served as the "Director of Dances" at the King's Theatre, Haymarket, from 1758 to 1763.[34] In his treatise Gallini drew connections between the body, the soul, and nature. The soul, acted upon by impulses derived from nature, found its outward expression in the body; the dancer studied shapes and gestures perfectly composed to draw pictures of the sentiments. "In Dancing," Gallini writes, "the attitudes, gestures, and motions derive ... their principle from nature, whether they caracterise joy, rage, or affection, in the bodily expression respectively appropriated to the different affections of the soul."[35] The dancer's body expressed universal truths and harmonies. The solo dancer created pictures; groups of dancers were composed into pleasing and instructive tableaux.

Training was required to increase flexibility and to encourage control of the musculature. Repetition was emphasized as the master put the student through exercises multiple times. In his *Theoretical and Practical Treatise on Dancing* (published in Naples in 1779), the late-eighteenth-century dancing master Gennaro Magri described, for instance, the execution of the *battements*, or "beating of the foot." The step involved beating one foot against the other on the ground or in a jump, and also referred to the lifting (raising or "beating") of one leg into the air.[36] By repeated practice, and the perfecting of this step, Magri insisted, it was possible to be a "perfect *ballerino*": "Whoever has not perfect use of the *battements* cannot be a *Ballerino*, because this, besides producing lightness of leg, looseness of sinews, and flexibility of the joints, gives a great softness and facility to any kind of detachment of the leg."[37] In training, the dancer would be required to practice the step as much as possible so the limbs would no longer feel heavy in this lifting or beating of the leg. When the dancer is out of practice, warned Magri ominously, "everything feels painful."[38]

Magri outlined the common perception that the property of equilibrium created the strongest and most perfect line in nature.[39] He defined equilibrium as a line that divided the body into two equal parts, descending from the center of the body to the base, where the feet were planted on the floor, with both feet equally turned outward from the knees and the hips.[40] This line of equilibrium, Magri said, helped to maintain the uprightness of the physical structure; in describing the line he drew from equivalencies in the world of science and architecture. While clearly this strongest and most perfect of lines was never to be fully achieved, the dancer's training encouraged a closer approach to this ideal: "This equilibrium has so much strength that the . . . whole world might be sustained on the point of a sewing needle, if it were possible. By force of equilibrium, those tall machines are supported, vast on top but standing on a slender base, to the wonder of spectators; and if the fine art of Architecture were joined to the most perfect equilibrium, and the earth were stable, never would such machines and buildings be liable to ruin."[41] Practice helped the dancer improve her balance with two feet on the floor, and also with one leg raised, in different directions around the body, at varying levels off the ground.[42]

Training in the mechanical aspects of dance demanded concentration, mental precision, and exactitude in attention to form. The dancer's mental energy was directed toward perceiving directions in space and creating patterns of physical geometry in imitation of what were held to be "naturally" symmetrical lines and arcs. The dancer's thought processes were always attuned to the measured precision of the music that invariably accompanied movement. From their earliest associations with court and ballroom, the various dance types were inseparable from their musical designations: the *chaconne, passacaille, minuet,* and *gigue* had comparable musical forms, each with its own particular meters and tempi. The dancer worked to execute dance steps within the given time and phrasing of the musical measures. The most skillful dancer, like the most gifted musician, could "play" with the rules—improvising within tightly designated boundaries—of phrasing, accent and dynamics. In his chapter entitled "Cadence," Magri defined this important element of the dance as the effort to fit movement to musical phrase, the striving toward a perfect timing of steps to music. According to their metric composition, the dance types neatly corresponded to two primary feeling states: lively dances (including the *gigue, gavotte, allemande*) were composed in duple meter, or binary time; the more stately and sedate dances (including the *chaconne, follia, amabile*) were those composed in triple meter, or ternary time.

While Magri brilliantly documented the technical standards of the ballet class, Jean-George Noverre's greatest contribution lay in his emphasis on the dancer's capacity to express through arm movements and facial gestures. Like Magri, Noverre analyzed the dance class and assessed common anatomical defects. He too believed that through "moderate but regular exercise" begun in childhood, the dancer learned to attain shapes that were strong, clear, and visually pleasing.[43] But it was the expressive component of dance that, for Noverre, raised the ballet to the status of high art, equivalent to that of grand opera or tragic drama.

Noverre addressed many of the artistic and philosophical debates of his time. His biographer, Deryck Lynham, writes that Noverre's "aesthetic theory, as expressed in his *Lettres sur la danse et sur les ballets*, published in 1760 . . . is that held by the enlightened aesthetes of his century."[44] Though ballet masters such as John Weaver (1673–1760), Jean Baptiste de Hesse (1705–79), Franz Anton Hilverding (1710–68), Gaspare Angiolini (1731–1803), Jean Dauberval (1742–1806), Maximilien (1741–87), Pierre Gardel (1758–1840), and Salvatore Vigano (1769–1821) were adamant that ballets should be expressive vehicles, organized as coherent theatrical works, it was Noverre who devoted years of his life to revising, editing, and publishing, in multiple volumes, his vision for the creation of the full-length *ballet d'action*.

Arguing for the elimination of the traditional use of masks, he declared that the face should be allowed to express dramatic truth: "A man's face is the mirror of his passions, in which the movements and agitations of the soul are displayed, and in which tranquillity, joy, sadness, fear and hope are expressed in turn."[45] And, he wrote, it was in this realm—which involved the soul's expression—that female dancers excelled. Female dancers hid the difficulties and strain involved in executing complicated dance steps with greater elegance than did men. Noverre wrote to an assumed male readership:

Why have women, who are naturally less sinewy, less muscular and less strong than we, have tender and voluptuous, lively and animated expressions, even when their muscles which co-operate in their movements are in a condition of unnatural strain? How, then, do they acquire that art which conceals labour, which hides bodily stress, and substitutes the most delicate and tender expressions for the grimaces born of the exertions put forth? The reason is that they pay particular attention to their exercises; they realise that a contortion disfigures the beauty of the face and changes its expression. They realise that the face is, as I have said, that part of us in which all expression is concentrated, and which is the faithful mirror of our feelings, movements and affections. Hence they put more soul, more expression and more interest into their work than men.[46]

The apparent difference in the physical structures, degrees of strength, and flexibility between the male and the female dancer similarly distinguished the nature of the dance vocabulary that it was possible for each to utilize. Men, it was believed, had the stronger limbs and greater range, while women "naturally" shaped their movements with greater attention to concepts of beauty and elegance. Noverre indicated that women's long skirts could hide a "multitude of sins," but, he said, expert dance observers could perceive faults even in spite of such coverings. Paintings and engravings of Baccelli in her dance costumes show that her skirts are slightly shorter than was conventional for street wear—they hit her at the base of her calf, slightly above her ankle—and that her dancing shoes, though heeled, are lighter and more flexible than the heavier and higher heels fashionable among many women in the 1770s and 80s.[47]

Elegant day and evening wear for ladies of wealth and high society was not designed to accommodate physical comfort, and wearing such restrictive dress with regularity may have conditioned female dancers to move and dance gracefully in spite of exerting great physical effort. Just prior to the French Revolution, fashionable aristocratic women adopted monumental hair styles that they wore powdered for formal occasions and unpowdered in everyday life.[48] Typically, too, women used white facial powder, which created the appearance of pale fragility. The dress dictated the movements a woman executed as part of her everyday existence and affected her automatic physical patterns of motion, thus shaping her dancing body. Women were used to the swinging of panniers as they maneuvered those wide understructures through doors or crowds. An upper-class woman customarily tilted her large headdress to enter a coach or sedan chair just as she sank into seats to accommodate her voluminous skirts. By the 1780s, the panniers began to shrink in size; waistlines rose higher, pushing the breast upward and thus requiring the deft application of kerchiefs, scarves, and fichus to hide and yet subtly expose portions of flesh. Theatrical costumes had been considerably lightened and shortened earlier in the eighteenth century; nevertheless, the expertise of the female dancer would have consisted in part in her smooth and elegant deployment of bodices and dresses, while maintaining a serene countenance and an elegant ease of movement.

Baccelli and Vestris were among the talented dancers who helped to shape the direction of the ballet of the late eighteenth century, training throughout their careers to marry virtuosity with dramatic expression and mime. The tension between those dancers who strove to accomplish more pirouettes, more beats, and longer balances and those who held that such "acrobatic tricks" lessened the aesthetic and moral value of the art form defined the greatest debate of their professional careers. The concern was real, for many dance lovers regretted that ballet was widely considered nothing more than a charming and amusing diversion. Some writers and commentators feared the tendency toward acrobatic spectacle would make the ballet all the more frivolous and insubstantial.

These ideas were not new to the eighteenth century, however, for tensions between technical prowess and artistic expression can be found in, for instance, the late seventeenth-century critiques of Abbé Michel de Pure. In his *Idée des spectacles anciens et nouveaux* (1688), de Pure alleged that the erosion of the glorious ballet embodied by *Le roi soleil* began even prior to Louis XIV's retirement from the stage in 1669 or 1670. De Pure lamented that dancing masters could not fulfill their choreographic ideas while dependent on the amateur dancing skills of their noble patrons. The late seventeenth-century move toward professionalism in dance, according to the art and dance historian Sarah Cohen, served to advance "the illusion of 'aristocratic' accomplishment," making it possible for professional dancers to teach and reproduce the "image of the noble body."[49] With this transformation of the art form, and with skilled professional bodies reproducing the illusion of nobility, dancers trained to perform increasingly intricate body movements, and dancing masters simultaneously brought out their developing technical abilities in performance.

As the eighteenth century progressed, dancers continued to experiment with greater levels of virtuosity even while the emphasis on theatrical coherence decreased. Lynham notes that while the comedy-ballets of Molière and the operas of Lully demonstrated significant theatrical integration, such close collaboration and unified vision was "lacking in the later ballets."[50] By 1730, the cynical prediction of Campra, primary composer of ballet music in Paris, that "the only way to popularize opera-ballet is to lengthen the dances and shorten the dancers' skirts," had been realized, for in that year Marie Camargo did indeed shorten "her skirt by several inches to just above the instep, the better to beat her *entrechats*."[51] Challenging other dancers of the early eighteenth century with her bold jumps and turns, Camargo stimulated both female and male virtuosity. Later in the century, Noverre's voluminous writings criticized the trend toward increasing virtuosity and vehemently protested ballet's status as mere entertainment. Noverre and other aesthesticians feared the tide was sweeping dance toward diversion and spectacle and away from more profound depictions of the human condition.

Throughout the eighteenth century, however, audiences were diversifying economically and growing larger.[52] Many of these viewers were not interested in opera and sought alternatives to the aristocratic *danse noble*. They demanded different kinds of entertainment, including spectacles that appealed to the eye and relied less on classical themes and allusions. Newly moneyed audiences encouraged the development of visually pleasing ballets that exploited virtuosity and eschewed the serious themes of opera and tragedy. Change was in the air, for novel approaches to theater production made such appealing spectacles possible. Innovations were widely disseminated in spite of the intricate system of *privilèges* that regulated the types of entertainment permissible at each theater in Paris. These *privilèges* delimited the nature of what could be presented at fairground theaters from those works produced at the Opéra.[53]

But ideas and invention could not be halted even by the guardians of tradition at the Opéra. Interchange between artists flourished and new mechanical inventions were developed. Innovations born in the seedier, lower-class boulevard theaters often seeped into the more refined opera houses. Dancers maintained a fluid passage between one theater and another. Frequently Opéra artists were hired to perform in the fairgrounds, while other dancers got their start in the minor theaters and eventually moved on to work at the Opéra, as did Noverre, who, early in his career, learned the tools of his trade in the provincial and boulevard theaters.

In 1776, at the end of his contract with the Viennese court, Noverre arrived in Paris, where, with the support of his former pupil, Marie Antoinette, now queen of France, he assumed the coveted post of ballet master at the Paris Opéra.[54] While Noverre had long sought the position, his tenure there was marred by friction. To the mighty dance establishment of the Paris Opéra, Noverre represented "the foreigner, the little impostor from the provinces, the reformer of the dance who would want to impose his ideas and upset established and easy going traditions." For the members of that establishment, Lynham says, Noverre became "a focal point for their venom."[55]

As the political intrigue and rivalries in Paris threatened to overtake him, Noverre did not renew his contract, and in 1781 he was only too glad to leave the lofty Opéra for a position at London's King's Theatre, Haymarket. The opportunity to work with Noverre, as well as the lucrative fees offered in London, prompted a number of fine dancers, including Pierre Gardel, Mademoiselle Théodore, and Louis Nivelon, to join Noverre in accepting contracts at the Haymarket. The dancers already in London who joined Noverre's troupe were all French trained though they had not grown up in the Opéra. These dancers included Antoine Bournonville, Simon Slingsby (an English dancer), and "that Italian ballerina of stunning beauty and elegance whom young Vestris had partnered the season before, Giovanna Baccelli."[56]

Londoners were excited by the arrival of foreign artists and anticipated the première of Noverre's new *ballet d'action*. The *Morning Herald and Daily Advertiser* for November 14, 1781, reported, "This year we are to have the first night, two Ballets, composed by the famous Noverre, and danced by Gardel, the first dancer in Paris, the first country in the world for dancing; Baccelli[,] the most favorite dancer that ever appeared in England, and Mad. Theodore, who stands without rival in the demi-character; besides Nivelon, who disputes the point of excellence with young Vestris."

The preparation of Noverre's new ballet would take more rehearsal time, however, and the newspaper article urged patience as its première was to be delayed. But the ballet Noverre offered as an alternative would hint at the fine work to come, according to the writer:

> Mr. Noverre's intention, as may naturally be supposed, was to have opened the theatre with one of those grand ballets which have established his reputation on the Continent on the firmest basis; but, lest the proprietors should be hurt, or the public disappointed by a longer delay, which must have been the consequence of greater preparations, he has chearfully consented to begin with a dance, which, tho' got up in a very superior style, may only be considered as an earnest of what the public are to expect from that gentleman's abilities, of which the town has already seen a sample in his ballet of *Medea and Jason*. The dances we allude to, are a *divertissement* of serious and demi-character, and a tragi-pantomime ballet, intituled [*sic*], *Les amans réunis,* or the Lovers reunited.

Since it was safe to assume many newspaper readers in London were novices in their appreciation of French ballet, the writer insisted on Noverre's vast importance in the world of dance: "Few people rightly understand the real meaning of ballet-master; in the true acceptation of the world, he is a man who, at the courts of foreign princes, is deemed capable of giving sumptuous fetes and entertainments. Therefore to say of one, as of Monsieur Noverre, that he is ballet-master to the Emperor, implies, that he is a person of refined taste, and most profound skill in his profession."

In England, no royal academy had ever been established to maintain the standards of dance technique, nor was there a tradition of training in the *danse noble* style, as there was in Paris. Without the intricate network of privileges, the English theaters, once they emerged from the dampening effects of Puritanism, were established on commercial and highly competitive grounds, and foreign superstars like Baccelli were almost universally preferred to the home-grown, home-trained English dancers with English names. In England it was assumed that ballet was a foreign import—that it was, in a word, French. Despite the notorious antipathy between the English and their French neighbors, Londoners responded with enthusiasm to the virtuoso dancers arriving on their shores.

Ballet in late eighteenth-century London was primarily a foreign import. It was also a male purlieu. The male predominance was noted in a commentary in the January 12, 1781, *Morning Herald and Daily Advertiser:* "Vestris, who since his appearance on the King's theatre, has proved more beneficial to the proprietors, than all the *A's* and *I's* of Italy [opera] could have done, has brought about a revolution very little expected. The Operas are now looked upon as a mere accessary [*sic*] to the dancing part of the entertainment, and that music alone attended to, which proclaims the approach of the capering hero." In January 1786, Lady Mary Coke wrote a letter breathlessly describing her visit to the opera, which had substantially less audience appeal than the dancing of Vestris: "This evening I went to the Opera but I can't give a good account of a bad thing some of the music is pretty but the Opera is sillier than any I ever heard and the performers are not too good, but Vestris, is if possible better than ever tis a pleasure to see dancing in such perfection tis pity there is no Woman that approaches his excellence to dance with him."[57]

But in the decades of the 1770s and 80s, if any woman could challenge the supremacy of Auguste Vestris on the London stage, it was certainly Giovanna Baccelli. The *Morning Herald and Daily Advertiser* reported on July 6, 1781:

> The connoisseurs in operatical exhibitions say, that Madame Baccelli's performance on the last night of the Vestris, exceeded any thing that has been seen there since the days of [German-born ballerina Anna] Heinel, to whom she proved herself the very first competitor, if not an entire equal. She exerted herself amazingly; and was received with as many, and as warm plaudits, as even the capering deities [Gaétan and Auguste Vestris] themselves, tho' that was the last night of their gracing this country with their performance.

To be sure, Londoners loved "their" Baccelli. On November 24, 1781, the *Morning Herald* called on the public to appreciate the technical virtuosity and refined grace of the Italian-born ballerina and her French partner, Pierre Gardel:

> Tho' serious dancing [*danse noble*] does not seem to take so much with public as the demicharacter and comic, yet it receives such additional merit from the amazing powers of Mons. Gardel and the inimitable graces of the Baccelli, that is likely to become a very great favorite; and is indeed already so with those who know that the execution of serious dancing is infinitely more difficult and demands much superior powers and judgment than are required in the demicharacter and comic. A slight attention to the movements of Gardel and Baccelli, will render this truth obvious, and consequently excite the admiration of all lovers of true excellence in graceful dancing.

Throughout her career, Baccelli was acclaimed for her graceful "serious," "grave" (also known as "noble") style of dancing. In her 1782 debut at the Paris Opéra, French audiences were struck by her musicality and technical skill. Although she initially encountered some French partisanship and jealous competition, Baccelli was able to win over most of her critics. "At one moment in her *pas* in *Electre*," says Ivor Guest, "she startled even the most hard-hearted spectators 'by standing on the toe of her foot without losing any of the grace and nobility which the style of the dance requires.' Another description, seemingly by the same hand, described her as 'alighting, standing and pirouetting on the toe.'"[58] Although, as Guest suggests, "It would be excessive to suggest that these two quotations amount to early evidence of *pointe* work," they certainly foretell the development of a technique that would feature the lightness and ethereality so desirable in ballerinas of the Romantic era. But, as Guest puts it, "Baccelli was no doubt dancing in heeled shoes, in which it may have been possible for a dancer with strong toes to rise momentarily onto the very tip."[59]

As a "serious" dancer, Baccelli executed "strong" and "soft" movements of the arms; she defined her space with smooth and fluid movements of legs and torso. The serious style required her to portray noble, dignified characters and demanded that through her use of focus, inclinations of the head, and arm gestures, she would command the stage space. She carved out the space through movements that remained *terre-à-terre* (that is, low to the ground, with very few jumps), but which created the effect of gracefulness and languor.[60] The dance historian Edmund Fairfax notes that "however easy and simple in appearance, the grave style demanded remarkable control on the part of the dancer in order to do justice to its predominantly slow, smooth movement. It was not without its own brilliance, for quick beats of different kinds provided contrast, together with a limited use of beaten jumps, such as entrechats."[61]

Again like Auguste Vestris, however, Baccelli was able to transcend the separations between genres; in some of her most popular roles, she was also described as an excellent *demi-caractère* dancer. Her roles in the *demi-caractère* style, such as that in *Les amans surpris,* were characterized by nimbleness, lightness, and speed. Fairfax quotes Giovanni Gallini's *A Treatise on the Art of Dancing* (1762), which characterizes the *demi-caractère* style as requiring lightness, nimbleness, and high, brilliant jumps: "In the half-serious stile [*sic*] we observe vigor, lightness, agility, brilliant springs, with a steadiness and command of the body. It is the best kind of dancing for expressing the more general theatrical subjects. It also pleases more generally."[62] Baccelli's *demi-caractère* roles included deities, idealized shepherdesses, or lighthearted characters from daily life.[63] Like Vestris, Baccelli strove in her training to assimilate a range of dance styles, and both she and Vestris embodied a late eighteenth-century melding of styles that would cohere further in the nineteenth century.

In spite of newspaper and eye-witness accounts, it remains difficult to know what Baccelli experienced as she danced. In speculating on Baccelli's probable dancing experience, I draw from the libretto of a ballet that was popularly associated with Baccelli, the Maximilien Gardel version of *Ninette à la cour.* A description of the ballet's plot exists in a ballet scenario (a *livret*) housed at the Bibliothèque de l'Opéra in Paris. The *livret* details a ballet-pantomime in three acts and five scenes, first staged for the royal court at Choisy on September 13, 1777, and at the Paris Opéra in August 1778.

Ivor Guest points out that in this work, one of the first significant efforts to integrate movement and mime, it was helpful that audiences might already have known the story. According to Guest, the origins of the ballet go back to a 1755 *opéra comique* version by Charles-Simon Favart, called *Le caprice amoureux, ou Ninette à la cour,* which was itself a parody of an earlier opera by Ciampi. The Gardel production at Choisy featured Gaétan Vestris as the King, Anna Heinel as the Countess, Pierre Gardel as Fabrice, Charles Dauberval as Colas, and Marie-Madeleine Guimard as Ninette. If the narrative originally held any subversive social messages, the ballet itself was charming and lighthearted and clearly intended to amuse and entertain audiences.

According to the *livret,* the first scene involves a group of celebratory peasants, including the lovers Colas and Ninette, who rejoice at their approaching marriage. The king and his hunting party next take the stage, and the king reveals to his companion, Fabrice, that he is in love with the peasant girl, Ninette. When Ninette dances out of her cottage, the king proposes she come to court with him. At that moment Colas arrives on the scene and, suspecting that Ninette is being unfaithful, launches into an argument with her. Angered, the now peevish Ninette refuses to make up with Colas and decides to leave with the king.

The second act shows Ninette in a palatial boudoir at court, where she examines her new courtly dress with amusement. Her ornate gowns hamper her movement and she finds herself tripping over her panniers. She is given diamonds with which to adorn herself, and she reacts with astonishment to their shining brilliance. Suddenly catching sight of a colorful bouquet, she drops the diamonds and runs to gather the bunch of flowers. Realizing that the beautiful flowers are artificial, she tosses them aside in disdain. A dancing master then arrives to instruct her in dance steps and courtly decorum. He proceeds to lead her through the minuet and the contredanse, an effort that proves disastrous as Ninette continually tips over from the weight of her heavy gown. Since she is clearly unable to move through the stately and courtly dances, the dancing master decides instead to try teaching her the fine art of flirting with a fan. Her response to this instruction is simply to yawn behind her fan at the king's arrival.

The countess, the king's betrothed, is distressed that her fiancé is once again dallying with a young peasant girl. At a ball that evening she taunts the king for his choice of a coarse peasant girl and proceeds to amuse herself at Ninette's expense. The scene shifts again to Ninette's boudoir in the palace, which Colas enters, still feeling angry with Ninette. When Ninette returns to the boudoir, dressed in her ball finery, Colas does not recognize her although he does respond to her flirtations, taking her hand and catching her as she pretends to swoon. When Ninette suddenly removes her veil, Colas is caught in his apparent act of betrayal—a flirtation with one he believes to be a fine lady of the court. Meanwhile, in her distress over Ninette's presence at court, the countess is next seen offering the king the opportunity to break off their engagement. Guiltily asserting that he has all the time remained faithful to his fiancée, he renews his commitment to the countess. He leaves her, sunken into a chair in her sadness and disbelief, where Ninette finds her. She reveals to the countess her desire to leave the court and return home to her true beloved, Colas. Just then, hearing the king arrive, Ninette bids the countess to hide. Unseen by all the others, Colas also arrives on the scene, and conceals himself. As Ninette extinguishes the lights in her chamber, the king declares his love to the countess, believing she is Ninette, while Colas reveals his love to Ninette, believing she is the countess. As might be expected, all is cleared up when torches are brought to illuminate the scene and both true couples (in their socially appropriate pairs) are reunited. The third act shows a fête in the gardens of the court, where the king blesses the young lovers and proceeds to renew his pledges to the countess.

Gaétan Vestris staged his own production of *Ninette à la cour* in London, a version based on the ballet-pantomime by Gardel, though Vestris, in typical eighteenth-century fashion, does not mention the earlier ballet or its creator. In the Vestris version, Ninette was performed by Giovanna Baccelli, who received kudos in the *Morning Herald and Daily Advertiser* on February 26, 1781, for her portrayal of the *demi-caractère* role:

> The grand ballet was danced in full perfection. The two Vestris acquitted themselves in a manner that seemed to surpass even the great expectations they had raised. We wish it were in the power of words to do ample justice to Madamoiselle Baccelli, whose part in the ballet was the more dificult as she was obliged to dance with that characteristic aukwardness [*sic*] which could not but sit uneasy on so accomplished a dancer. The ballet has undergone some judicious alterations, and we are of opinion that it might yet be curtailed without any detriment to the performance.

A 1783 poem from the pen of the French dance enthusiast M. Duplain describes the ballerina Madeleine Guimard (1743–1816) in the part. The poem sheds some light on the ballet that audiences would have seen and the dancing that Baccelli would have experienced.[64] Duplain's poem traces a woman's body moving in space and her embodiment of the dance steps, as well as the gestures and feelings appropriate to the depiction of individual characters. Duplain's association of the *danseuse* Guimard with a goddess is a conventional eighteenth-century poetic trope, but his movement description is useful. His account suggests that for observers of the day, the finest dancers appeared to move fully through space, and that these dancers' physical investment in executing movement phrases seemed both rich and full-bodied.

Today, the eighteenth-century dancing body inevitably seems restricted by costume and sharply delineated spatial pathways, and it appears to be cut off from free-flowing, weighty movement. But dance lovers of the late eighteenth century perceived something quite distinct. These viewers sought legibility—clarity and balance—in relatively static but visually pleasing positions and figure groupings. They looked for verticality and clarity of execution and expected to encounter issues of Nature versus Art. To the late eighteenth-century viewer, a dancer's "naturalness" was proportional to her elegance, and her ease resulted from the "art" of her expert training.

Duplain writes, "Quelle Divinité lui prête sa ceinture, / Rend son jeu *naturel*, & pare la *Nature?*" Guimard, says Duplain, displays an ease in her torso that belies the intricacy of her quickly moving feet: "Son buste *harmonieux* n'offre rien que d'*aise*. / Que ses pieds distraits ont bien leur simpathie!" Guimard is described as challenging verticality, giving an illusion of abandonment and seeming to cast herself into the full sweep and flow of movement. The viewer responds to the kinesthetic illusion of her physical freedom, while sensing that the dancer's graceful, trained body remains ever in control: "Abandonner son corps sans perdre l'équilibre, / Choisir un point central & courir au hazard, / S'élever avec goût, retomber avec art."

Dance audiences of the day watched artists express a range of emotions. In their view, a dancer's range was evoked in the variety and vividness of her gestures and facial expressions. In the *Cadre troisième,* Duplain describes Guimard's portrayal of a youthful, happily carefree girl in her childlike smiles and bright, cheerful gestures of innocence. When, in the course of the ballet's narrative, this naive character is confronted by evil, Guimard's eyes, face, and trembling, unsteady movements express her character's fear and desperation.[65] Her flirtatious vivacity is evident in the character of Ninette, in the ballet that won Baccelli many accolades. As Ninette, Guimard's playful teasing of her lover Colas is offset, says Duplain, by the delicate, sweet smile that plays across her lips: "Un souris délicat qui pénètre & qui touche."[66]

The delicate, sweet smile described by Duplain is also revealed in a lithograph representing Giovanna Baccelli dancing in Louis Simonet's 1781 production of *Les amans surpris.* Simonet's work was first produced in London at the King's Theatre on December 6, 1780, and received twenty-two performances during the 1781–82 season; in June 1786 it was revived and that season received five performances. Baccelli's performance in this ballet attracted Gainsborough's attention, as was noted earlier, and it was the role through which Baccelli purportedly achieved a sensational popularity.[67] The lithograph, by J. Thornwaite after James Roberts, depicts Baccelli in her costume for her role: her bell-like skirt is hooped, and it is shortened to midcalf.[68] Baccelli's face is shown in profile, a view distinguished by her long, slender nose. The dancer is shown holding a garland of roses, other flowers, and greenery. Wearing low-heeled slippers, she steps onto half-toe, *demi-pointe,* on her left foot; with her right foot raised slightly behind, she appears to have been caught in the middle of a *demi-coupé.* Her head is turned to the right and the bow of her bonnet hangs from her chin, bisecting the front of her bodice. The lithograph presents an idealized picture and emphasizes her tiny waist, her upright carriage, and her grace and symmetry in suspension. The bouffant skirt heightens the sense of her lightness, balanced by her poise, stability, and serenity. With eyes modestly downcast, she glances over her right arm rather than at the viewer. The slight smile that plays across her lip suggests delicacy and charm. It is the same slight smile that all of her portraitists managed to convey.

I speculate that Baccelli's most salient features as an artist were her vivacity and graceful proficiency, along with her physical beauty and charm. She was a highly trained dancer in the noble French style and her expertise was seen to best advantage in the clarity of her brilliant technique. Although she was noted in the elegant noble style, she was clearly able to win the hearts of her English audiences in her light-hearted and virtuosic portrayal of Ninette. Baccelli's attention to technique combined concentrated effort, discipline, focused attention to line, clarity and serenity of execution, rhythm and musicality, breath and expression. Free to move within these bounds, Baccelli never danced without a decorous constraint and limitation. Her dance vocabulary emphasized play within the boundaries set by an academic *danse d'école*, any fluidity and weightiness held in check by the attention to principles of verticality and line. Baccelli's vivacious personality and the sparkling nature of many of her roles and characters might have prompted her to push just to the limits of proportion and modesty. But, restrained by her corset and heavy skirts, Baccelli never completely released her weight into gravity or outward into space. Exciting her spectators with her physical beauty and her seductive playfulness as well as with her great control and acumen, Baccelli danced with fleet, delicate steps in clearly etched patterns through space, her face always expressive and alive.

Given her technical refinement and ease in virtuoso movement as well as her established place in the hearts of British audiences, it is paradoxical that during Noverre's tenure as dancing master at the King's Theatre Baccelli's place on the stage was less prominent than might have been expected. She was frequently seen in secondary roles while Madame Simonet, a dancer of lesser reputation, was given leading parts.[69] As a former pupil of Noverre, Simonet may have displayed the acting skills he tried to develop, and he highlighted her abilities in spite of Baccelli's technical expertise. In *Rinaldo and Armida*, for instance, Noverre selected Simonet to dance Armida while Théodore and Baccelli danced the spirits who distract the knights. In his *Adela of Ponthieu*, too, Simonet was Adela while Théodore, Crespi, and Baccelli danced incidental roles as ladies of the court. Nevertheless, Baccelli, like Vestris, developed as a dramatic performer so that by 1784, dancing in Venice, she was able to take on "the heavy rôle of Medea in Lefebvre's production of (Noverre's) *Giasone e Medea*."[70]

Theater records at the Fondazioni Cini in Venice document that Baccelli performed in that city during the 1783–84 Carnevale season, though few other accounts seem to have survived. Ivor Guest describes an incident during her first performance in Venice, in which Baccelli was greeted with the loud disapproval of the Italian audience. A recognized ballerina who had been applauded by audiences in London and Paris, she first encountered hostility and catcalls from the partisan spectators at the city's principal theater, Teatro San Benedetto. The intercession of her stage manager and of her patronness, Cecilia Zen Tron, had the desired effect and Baccelli was later recognized with warmth by the Venetian audiences.[71]

Some newspaper accounts document Baccelli's appearances in 1788–89 at Teatro San Benedetto. Reviews in the *Gazzetta Urbana Venetia* suggest that this time, Baccelli's reputation preceded her and that she was greeted in Venice with great acclaim as a recognized and esteemed artist. She is both powerful and graceful, according to the review appearing in the *Gazzetta Urbana Venetia* on January 21, 1789. On February 7, 1789, the same newspaper duly praised her widespread acclaim and declared it well merited. One week later the *Gazzetta* reviewer called her the "celebre Signora Baccelli" (the celebrated Madmoiselle Baccelli).[72]

The *Gazzetta* writer on January 28, 1789, spoke highly of a new ballet in which its creator, the ballet master Francesco Clerico, had skillfully combined movement and pantomime. The reviewer praised Clerico's invention of beautiful figures and the artistry with which he deployed groups of dancers on the stage. The work's beauty was only enhanced, wrote this reviewer, by its rich and magnificent costumes and ornaments, and by the performances of a highly talented company of dancers, among whom the "incomparable" Mademoiselle Baccelli and the "graceful" Signor Angiolini were singled out. After their first dance of the evening, the couple apparently surprised their audience by executing another simple but lovely and expressive *pas de deux*, and the writer was particularly enchanted with Baccelli's ability to make difficult dance vocabulary appear both elegant and easy. "The highest quality of Mad. Baccelli is to perform the most difficult operations in dance with an ease and confidence to make them seem easy, [thus] concealing the [required] effort."[73]

Other reviews in the *Gazzetta Urbana Venetia* from early 1789 shed light on Baccelli's particular artistry. One writer was particularly impressed by Baccelli's expertise in roles in the *demi-caractère* style, reporting, "The inimitable Mad. Baccelli forms [is] the delight of the most refined [artistic] tastes, with the exactness, the levity, the precision and the strength with which her beautiful operations [gestures] are executed in that half-noble character in which she is singular and excellent."[74] But Baccelli also received kudos for her great versatility, as at the end of the Carnevale season she was to dance a "capriccio," or a "pot-pourri" of lively dances to the accompaniment of popular songs:

> The untiring genius of the celebrated Mad. Baccelli, together with the most honest zeal of the advantages of the Company she serves, made her invent a "ballabile" piece that in France would be called a Pot-Pourri, and among us could be called a caprice adapted for the last days of Carnival, in which she will perform in dance certain modern popular songs, whose easy tunes are sung in the streets.
> The prodigious ability of this famous Ballerina, who overcomes any difficulties and can bend herself in all different ways, will make her obtain even in this [case] a full applause, moved by the admiration and by the pleasure, and by a certain playfulness that she diffuses with grace and liveliness, that accompany her difficult operations, which take . . . from her frankness and outmost expertise . . . an air of easy execution.[75]

Baccelli may occasionally have created her own dances, although the frequency with which she contributed her own work is hard to determine. Edmund Fairfax quotes several dancing masters, including Magri, Gallini, and Noverre, who indicate that the ballet dancer's "invention" of dance steps and caprices was readily encouraged in the eighteenth century.[76] On at least one occasion, Venetian dance audiences were promised a solo of Baccelli's own invention. Unfortunately, in this case she was prevented from dancing the solo, newspaper accounts reveal, when the entire evening's performance was canceled as a result of an accident incurred by her partner, Signor Angiolini.[77]

Inevitably, there are gaps in the record: why and how frequently did Baccelli return to Venice? Did she choose to go for professional or personal reasons? What was her relationship to her wealthy noble patroness, the notoriously flirtatious Cecilia Zen Tron? For one thing, Venice during Carnevale undoubtedly promised excitement and magic. Carnevale, writes Alfonso Lowe, was "the quintessence of all that was light-hearted, frivolous, carefree and vicious."[78] Cecila Zen Tron was widely renowned for her gaiety, frivolity, and lax morality, and stories persist about her easy readiness to "give of her favors." Then, too, ballerinas in Venice were commonly reported to be sexually available. Even given the general abandonment of social codes during Carnevale, the "looseness of conduct among females," writes Lowe, "seems to have been mainly that of ballet dancers."[79] Maurice Andrieux also describes the notoriety of dancers, writing that ballerinas were known to have "led brazen lives" and that many were "obvious prostitutes."[80]

The Venetian stage was clearly an alluring and intriguing environment, but did it also present professional rewards for Bacelli? It seems likely. At Teatro San Benedetto, Baccelli had opportunities to take on a different and no doubt challenging set of roles, and she had the chance to perform ballets that she did not dance in London or Paris. In 1789 she danced in works by Clerico, including *Il ritorno d'Agamennone, I sacrifizi di Tauride* and *Il filosofo deriso,* and in ballets by Pietro Angiolini, including *Le due rivali.*

As an aging ballerina, however, Baccelli found her options were narrowing. Price, Milhous, and Hume explain, "Second dancers sometimes descended to the rank of *figurant* as they got older. Male dancers at all levels had the option of teaching; there is no evidence that women did so as a regular occupation, though individuals managed to teach on a small scale. If lesser women dancers helped in dancing schools, their names were not advertised."[81] There seems to be no indication that Baccelli ever taught dancing lessons, but an advertisement in the *Morning Herald and Daily Advertiser* for November 24, 1781, reveals that Baccelli's rival, Madame Simonet, the noted dramatic ballerina who performed the leading roles in many of Noverre's ballets, did take some female students. Madame Simonet sought to instruct ladies of nobility and gentry in the "graceful and elegant part of education," according to the advertisement. The same newspaper on January 22, 1785, refers to lessons taught by Madame Rossi, the wife (or mistress) of Charles le Picq, who was himself a dancing master and performer: "Madame Rossi begs Leave to inform the Nobility and Gentry that she continues as usual to instruct Ladies in the art of Dancing, both abroad and at her own house, No. 33 Pall-Mall, where she will give every information concerning the terms, days, and hours of attendance."[82]

Those women who, unlike Baccelli, lacked the support of a wealthy male protector during their postperformance years may have had to face the threat of poverty. The situation for the genuinely talented and beautiful female dancer—like Baccelli—who rose to star status was entirely distinct from that of the impoverished, native-born women who served as *figurantes.* These were young women who lacked substantial training in dance, but whose onstage roles required them to walk, assemble in poses, and carry stage properties. Most often they came from the ill-educated and neediest classes, whose prospects of early death from disease and hunger were not to improve throughout the nineteenth century.

THE BACCELLI LEGEND LINGERS

If the Duke of Dorset was more renowned for playing cricket than he was for his political or diplomatic skills, his correspondence dating from his ambassadorship nevertheless presents the picture of a man of the world, capable of conducting himself with grace and casual ease. He was also an art collector of catholic tastes, and for this we must be grateful. In part, impressions of Baccelli linger today because of the duke's fondness for her and his patronage of artists who represented her. Today's visitor to Knole is struck by this, for a tour of the house feels like a visit to a private and venerable art gallery. Touring the rooms that are open to the public, one encounters Locatelli's full-length sculpture of the nude Baccelli on her couch. The sculpture has been returned to public view after Dorset's wife, Arabella Cope, ordered it banished to the basement, and it now has a place at the foot of the Great Staircase, where light filters through small panes of leaded glass and plays over her shapely body. Baccelli reclines in regal nonchalance. She has propped herself up on her elbows on top of pillows decorated with long tassels. The sheets at the bottom of the couch are gracefully but casually rumpled. Baccelli's hair is piled high and loose, informally; one stray ringlet dangles enticingly around her neck. As in other portraits and lithographs, Baccelli's face is distinctive for its long, elegant nose. Her fleeting, delicate smile visibly softens the sculpted stone. It is the same slight smile that Reynolds saw and that Gainsborough captured in the portrait that hangs at the Tate. These artworks hint at the mystery of the woman and the luster of the ballerina. They give life to the Baccelli legend.

2

ADÈLE
DUMILÂTRE

THÉOPHILE GAUTIER, the romantic poet, novelist, the-
ater critic, and ballet enthusiast, appreciated the creation of beauty onstage.[1]
For him, nothing was more beautiful or more artful than the idealized female
body moving through the *pas*, attitudes, gestures, and leaps of the nineteenth-
century ballet vocabulary. When Gautier watched Adèle Dumilâtre dance as
Myrtha, the queen of the Wilis, in the first performance of *Giselle*, for which
he wrote the libretto, he was struck by her virginal allure. Describing the
opening of the ballet's second act, Gautier writes, "The reeds part and there
come into view, first, a little twinkling star, then a crown of flowers, then two
beautiful blue eyes, looking gently startled and set in an oval of alabaster, and
then finally the whole of that lovely form—slender, chaste, graceful, and worthy of Diana of old—that we know as Adèle Dumilâtre." Using metaphors
that defy the concrete, Gautier describes Dumilâtre's opening solo in terms
of weightlessness and mysterious nonphysicality. He continues, "With that
melancholy grace that is characteristic of her, she frolics in the pale starlight,
skimming across the water like a white mist, poising on the bending branches,
stepping on the stalks of the flowers like Virgil's Camilla who walked on the
corn without bending it, and with a wave of her magic wand summons her
subjects, the other wilis, who emerge in veils of moonlight from tufts of reeds,
clusters of shrubbery and blooms of flowers."[2]

In a letter to Heinrich Heine that was published in *La Presse* on July 5, 1841, Gautier describes how he took his inspiration for the ballet's libretto from one of Heine's poems. Gautier writes about the creation of the ballet—its libretto a collaborative effort between himself and Vernoy de Saint-Georges, its choreography by Jean Coralli and Jules Perrot, and its music composed by Adolphe Adam. Gautier was infatuated with the newly prominent Italian ballerina Carlotta Grisi and dreamed up the role of Giselle for her, while her lover, the ballet master Perrot, created the major portions of her dancing. Essays and reviews from the period describe Grisi as a delicate but exuberant dancer and attest to the seminal importance of the ballet itself. But Adèle Dumilâtre remains less known. Who was this woman who first danced Myrtha, the icy counterpart to the forgiving, warm, and full-blooded Giselle?

The search for Adèle Dumilâtre sent me back though the mists of French romanticism to find the woman within the idealizing literature and iconography of the early nineteenth century. I came to see Adèle Dumilâtre in terms of the women she was not: not a front-ranking ballerina, she was a successful French-born ballerina of the second tier. Not the mother, wife, or daughter of a middle- or upper-class family, she was an ambitious, self-sufficient Parisian woman of the theater, whose career held her in opposition to the nineteenth-century women of bourgeois values. Though known for her chaste elegance onstage, Dumilâtre led the life of a professional dancer, which meant that off the stage she was a woman of ill-repute. In other words, she was all that a "good" middle-class woman was not. Her social status echoed the myths of the era itself, for romantic literature figuratively replays the trope of females in binary opposition to their sisters. Various nineteenth-century constructs make woman either a maid or a lady; a virgin or a whore; a fragile, poetic, and sensitive soul or a powerful, earthy, and sensual paramour.[3] The French ballet of the early nineteenth century, in resonance with the cultural and political mood of the time, recreated and reconfigured these polarities, characterizing its romantic ballerinas as either full-blooded and earthy, exemplified in the enormously popular character dances, or delicate and supernatural, represented in the *ballet-blanc*.[4] The realities of the dancers' lives, and their experiences as working women, however, were far more complex than the dyadic relationship pictured in novels and performances.

Mirroring the social structures of the day, the nineteenth-century Paris Opéra maintained its own internal hierarchies. Thus, Dumilâtre's professional stature served to distinguish her from hundreds of other muslin-clad *danseuses*. As a native-born French ballerina, Dumilâtre occupied some middle ground between the sheer penury of the impoverished French ballet girls—the starving little *rats* and *figurantes*—and the international acclaim of those romantic ballet superstars who, like Marie Taglioni (Italian), Fanny Elssler (Viennese), Carlotta Grisi (Italian), and Lucille Grahn (Danish), were not French-born. It can be difficult to get a sense of Dumilâtre as distinct from her many anonymous cohorts. She has been overshadowed by more famous ballerinas, and her story is often embedded within critiques of other female dancers. In one review, for instance, Gautier merely glances over her presence in his description of a *pas de trois* danced by Mademoiselle Albertine, mentioning the "charming" Adèle Dumilâtre "and her sister Sophie, who would be really pretty if only she had a little more nose."[5] One of a pair of real-life dancing sisters, Adèle nevertheless stepped out of the shadows of the romantic ballet as the more successful and, ultimately, more renowned of the two female Dumilâtres.

Offstage, ballerinas like Dumilâtre held an unacknowledged social station: they were both slightly disreputable and relatively well known. While most were "kept women," many were also hard workers, and some were ambitious to advance their careers. Unlike their counterparts in bourgeois households, nineteenth-century ballerinas, including Dumilâtre, held minor celebrity status and wielded some power in the market economy. They may have lacked the sanction of society and church, yet successful ballet dancers could shape their careers and plan for their retirements. Inhabiting a theatrical world whose magical effects were built out of tulle and gaslight, pointe shoes, corsets, machinery, and vapor, the romantic ballerina was a working woman of substantial autonomy and self-control.

As Dumilâtre stepped out of the clusters of other tutu-clad *danseuses* and into my range of vision, she began to distinguish herself as someone more real than symbolic, a woman rather than an idealized figure of purity or sensuality. Dumilâtre gradually emerged as a professional woman of talent, self-sufficiency, resolve, and discipline. From the 1830s, when she first danced in the *corps de ballet* at the Paris Opéra, until her retirement from the stage in 1848, Adèle Dumilâtre appears to have been a noted beauty and a hard-working, ambitious woman of the theater who was determined to advance in her career.

Born in Paris on June 30, 1821, Adèle was the younger of two sisters whose father had been an actor at the Comédie Française. In spite of her father's notion that Adèle might take to the dramatic stage, the girl's ballet teacher, Charles Petit, managed to convince him of her talents as a dancer, and little Adèle was destined for a career in ballet. Like the Baccelli family, the Dumilâtres were theater folk, and it was no doubt assumed Adèle and Sophie would support themselves—with supplementary protection from male "patrons," of course—as working women of the stage. Unlike many of the young girls who frequently took to dance as a means of escaping their desperately impoverished origins, the talented and strikingly handsome Adèle Dumilâtre soon emerged from anonymity. Père Dumilâtre was clearly determined that his daughters would be granted the recognition to which he believed they were entitled. According to Albéric Second, a man about town and journalist, an anecdote about the elder Dumilâtre's ambitious publicity campaign on behalf of his daughters made the rounds of backstage gossip. Second relates that seated in the audience at the Opéra one night, M. Dumilâtre, assuming the pose of a disinterested observer, remarked to a neighbor: "Ah, who is that charming young dancer?" "Why," the neighbor answered, "that is Mademoiselle Adèle Dumilâtre." "I thank you, sir," announced Père Dumilâtre to all within earshot, "how beautiful she is. There is truly no one as beautiful as she!" Then, when Sophie appeared on stage, there followed a similar question and response. "Ah," enthused the father, "there is no one so talented as she." But the identity of the questioner was inauspiciously revealed when a fellow actor declared, "Surely you know those young women, Père Dumilâtre! They are your daughters."[6]

Steadily rising through the ranks to the status of *première danseuse*, Dumilâtre in 1841 became one of the first dancers to replace Marie Taglioni in the title role of *La sylphide*.[7] She created the role of Myrtha in *Giselle* (1841) and, with the intervention of a male patron, was ultimately selected to take the lead role in Joseph Mazilier's *Lady Henriette* (1844). All the same, Dumilâtre had reason to compete for roles and be anxious about garnering her share of audience attention as the romantic ballet was dominated by ballerinas, many of whose names are legendary in dance history. As Alphonse Royer pointed out in his *Histoire de l'Opéra*, around the great stars like Taglioni, Elssler, Grisi, Cerrito, and Grahn (none of whom was French born) there gravitated a swarm of "charming" second-tier ballerinas distinguished by real talent who were less remarked upon. Among these Royer includes names such as Mesdemoiselles Dumilâtre and Duvernay, Madame Guy-Stéphan, and Mademoiselle Priora (all of whom were French).[8] Still, for those who had some measure of fame, there were engagements to be had. Like their counterparts in the eighteenth century, many nineteenth-century dancers traveled widely through Europe and America and even journeyed into Russia. Like other ballerinas, Dumilâtre accepted engagements abroad, making frequent visits to dance in London, where she was warmly received at Her Majesty's Theatre in 1843 and at the Theatre Royal in Drury Lane in 1844–45, while in 1846 she performed at La Scala in Milan.

Descriptions of Baccelli emphasized the eighteenth-century ballerina's elegance and her refined but powerful virtuosity. Dumilâtre, on the other hand, was noted for her alabaster skin and the limpid, ethereal quality of her movement. Benjamin Lumley, long-time director of Her Majesty's Theatre in London, recalled that Dumilâtre was the "incarnation of grace," and he presumed to cite her name alongside that of Marie Taglioni. Writing of the 1843 season at Her Majesty's, Lumley allowed that journalists of the day were struck by Dumilâtre's London debut in the divertissement *L'aurore*. "The *debutante* achieved a triumph, and was declared one of the effective representatives of the 'ideal' school of dancing (of which Taglioni was the head), in contradistinction to the 'realistic' school of Cerito [*sic*] and others."[9]

In her own day, Dumilâtre was a memorable ballerina, though she did not rank among the most renowned ballerinas of the Romantic era. A woman who, by most accounts, was of great physical beauty, she was also a gifted technician. Perhaps, though, it was her unusually tall stature and her air of reserved dignity that prohibited her from ascending to the upper echelon of ballerinas, alongside the non-French dance luminaries. Nevertheless, in the hands of a choreographic master like Jules Perrot, Dumilâtre's "chaste" elegance could be shown to its best advantage. Making her London debut in Perrot's minor divertissement called *L'aurore*, Dumilâtre achieved popular success. Guest writes, "Jules [Perrot] had done well by her in his choreography, showing off her strong technique and turning her unusual height to good advantage by devising passages that emphasised the natural elegance of her line."[10]

A print exists today of Dumilâtre in *L'aurore*, which Perrot choreographed to music by Pugni and which received its première at Her Majesty's Theatre in London in 1843.[11] In this picture an idealized figure floats on a bed of clouds above a small cluster of hills visible in the distance below. Across the horizon, the sun appears to be rising. Nestled in the clouds, the nymph reclines on her left hip and elbow; she is dressed in a wispy pink skirt that reaches to her midcalf. Her shapely legs and absurdly tiny slippered feet are crossed in front, as she lies in her delicate nest. The features that noticeably stand out are her unusually large eyes and the dark, soft hair that surrounds her oval face.

By 1848, however, Adèle Dumilâtre began to show signs of readiness to retire from the stage. Guest notes that the première of *Griseldis* was declared a triumph for the leading ballerina, Carlotta Grisi, and that the production itself was regarded as an all-around success. Nevertheless, critics reported that the leading male *danseur*, Lucien Petipa, was careless, while Dumilâtre, who took the leading rôle in the *fête des jardinières*, was disappointing. Charles Maurice complained of Dumilâtre's increasing feebleness and of the lack of vibrancy in her conventional smile.[12]

Dumilâtre apparently experienced little hardship when she ended her career. Castil-Blaze lists her as one of a number of female dancers who became wealthy and/or attained high social status after retirement. His list of those attaining prosperity and prestige includes some of the best known ballerinas: Marie Sallé, who retired in 1735, had become a millionaire; in 1778 Anne-Marguerite Dorival had achieved a large fortune; Fanny Elssler married a Prussian banker; and Adèle Dumilâtre became the Countess Drake del Castillo.[13] Indeed, it appears that Dumilâtre was fortunate, as Guest describes her retirement years this way: "For several years, Adèle Dumilâtre was the mistress of a rich landowner from Havana, but after she left the Opéra she married an equally wealthy gentleman by the name of Francisco Drake del Castillo. Being left a widow some years later, she then went to live with her sister Sophie at Pau, and later moved, with her two sons and daughter, to a château in Touraine. She died in Paris, at her home in the Rue Cler, on May 4th, 1909, shortly before her eighty-eighth birthday."[14] Even in retirement, though, Dumilâtre's image was not entirely effaced. Gautier noted that in an 1853 revival of *Giselle*, "we regretted the absence of Adèle Dumilâtre, that beautiful Queen of the Wilis, a moonbeam shaded with gauze."[15]

Since Baccelli's day, the ballet vocabulary continued toward a merging of the genres. Following upon the innovations of dancers like Vestris and Baccelli, *danseurs* and *danseuses* expanded their levels of virtuosity, blending the classic *danse d'école* with the more acrobatic *demi-caractère* styles. But there was also now an even greater distinction between the dance vocabulary of men and that of women. Lynn Garafola describes this gendering of the ballet in the early nineteenth century "that eventually transformed ballet into an art about women performed by women for men." Pointe work was the most visible demarcation; though it could have been practiced by men, it became "a uniquely female utterance." As pointe technique evolved from its eighteenth-century practitioners, it came to serve as "a metaphor for femininity—the Romantic ballet's true subject."[16]

Romantic ballet was about "woman"—celebrated for her sensual physicality and, paradoxically, also adored for her ethereal weightlessness. Concurrently, the stage at the Paris Opéra was notably bereft of men. For some observers, the loss of a starring male presence was palpable and tragic. Gone were the days of the great *danseurs nobles*, writers like Alphonse Royer noted with despair. Royer remarked on the progressive extinction of the male species at the Opéra and rued the passing of grand male dancers like Vestris, Louis Dupré, or Louis

Duport. The sole male dancer of excellence left to us, he declared, is Jules Perrot, who was born at the beginning of the century, studied under Auguste Vestris, and trained Carlotta Grisi and guided her to her eventual fame. But, with the exception of Perrot, "la danse des hommes a passé de mode," Royer writes. No longer fashionable, male dancers served only to support ballerinas, to prevent them from falling while they executed *arabesques penchées* or multiple perilous piroutes.[17] Castil-Blaze, too, noted the gender inequities, remarking on the passing of male dancers from the scene and the consequent preponderance of women in *travestie* roles.[18]

Garafola points out that "the disappearance of the male dancer coincided with the triumph of romanticism and marketplace economics," and that the phenomenon of the *danseuse en travestie* "invoked both the high poetic and the bordello underside of romantic and post-romantic ballet."[19] Further, she notes, "As an emblem of wanton sexuality, feminized masculinity, and amazon inviolability, the *danseuse en travestie* symbolized in her complex persona the many shades of lust projected by the audience on the nineteenth-century dancer."[20] Gautier, for one, could never pass up the opportunity to watch beautiful women display their legs in men's form-fitting *pantalons*. He praised Thérèse Elssler's arrangements of her sister Fanny's *pas* in her choreography for the 1838 ballet *La volière* because of its virtual exclusion of men. As choreographer and manager for Fanny, Thérèse—dancing *en travestie*—most often also partnered her sister. Gautier was pleased, he said, because Mademoiselle Thérèse had relieved audiences of the "tedium" of having to witness male performers. "Indeed there is nothing more disagreeable than a man showing his red neck, great muscular arms, parish beadle legs, and the whole of his heavy frame shuddering with leaps and pirouettes."[21]

But the crowning blow to the once noble male dancer was certainly rendered by the critic Jules Janin, who, in writing to a decidedly male readership, declared that "woman is the queen of ballet," and man is "useful accessory," the "shading in a painting," and the "green hedge that surrounds the flowers of the parterre." Janin wrote in an 1840 review of Perrot's ballet-opera, *Zingaro*,

> The *grand danseur* appears so sad, so heavy! He is at once so unhappy and so pleased with himself! He reacts to nothing, he represents nothing; he is nothing. Speak to me of a pretty dancing girl, who willingly offers her graceful airs and elegant figure, who shows us in such subtle ways all the treasures of her beauty. God have mercy, how wonderfully I understand that. I know exactly what to expect from this pretty person and am quite willing to follow wherever she leads in the sweet lands of love. But a man, a frightful man, as ugly as you or me, with an empty, vacant gaze, who capers aimlessly, a creature made

expressly to bear a rifle, saber, and uniform! That this being should dance like a woman, impossible! This bearded person, who is a community leader, and elector, a member of the municipal council, a man who ... appears before us in a sky blue satin tunic, a cap with a floating plume that amorously strokes his cheek—a frightful *danseuse* of the masculine sex who pirouettes center stage, while the pretty ballet girls repectfully keep their distance. Most certainly these *grands danseurs* are something impossible, intolerable, something made expressly to deny all our pleasures.[22]

In his 1860 publication *Letters on Dance and Choreography,* the French-trained Danish dancer, choreographer, and ballet master Auguste Bournonville commented on the changing status of men on the opera house stage. Written in Paris, these outspoken letters document Bournonville's observations and responses to the training and world of the Paris Opéra that both he and Dumilâtre would have known in the 1830s and 1840s. The letters are clearly modeled on, and partly an answer to, those published a century earlier by Jean-Georges Noverre. In his third letter, Bournonville, like Gautier and Janin, acknowledged the disappearance of the male dancer and the greater prominence now given to the role of the female *danseuse.*[23] The picture was different in the eighteenth century, Bournonville writes, for then "the reputation of the men was at least equal to that of the women; their success was naturally shared, since their energy, masculine elegance and polished schooling earned the audience's esteem for the *danseurs;* just as their flexibility, the *exquisite finish* of their execution, and their feminine grace, together with the heart's temptations, achieved, as they have always and everywhere, the triumph of the fair sex."[24] Marie Taglioni's arrival on the scene marked a dramatic change in the importance of the female dancer on stage, notes Bournonville. After Taglioni's phenomenal debut in *La sylphide,* the technical demands placed on the female dancer were substantially increased and ballet became all but synonymous with woman.

Taglioni's presence heralded a new era for she brought to the stage the appearance of innocence and youth. She bore no taint of voluptuousness or sensuality, but was "a real sylph, a daughter of the waves." Projecting his own imaginative conception of her ethereal purity, Bournonville recast Taglioni's life circumstances, avoiding references to her lovers and her occasional pregnancies. For Bournonville, Taglioni was "a virtuous maiden, a young lady of good family, in short everything that can be imagined as pure, gracious and poetic, combined with a talent whose outstanding quality was an airy lightness."[25]

Despite her peccadilloes, it was her symbolic purity that mattered to romantic audiences. When Marie Taglioni debuted in her father's 1832 ballet *La sylphide,* the image of the ballerina was suddenly and irrevocably altered.

Filippo Taglioni's ballet, Guest writes, was as "momentous a landmark in the chronicles of Romantic art as 'The Raft of the Medusa' and *Hernani*."[26] *La sylphide* marked a new direction in ballet's mood, atmosphere, and theme, and Marie Taglioni's appearance as the sylphide epitomized a distinctly different ideal for the ballerina, one that was made visible in the singular body of this rather unprepossessing ballerina, whose mystique and "virginal" grace paradoxically drove her audiences to near frenzies. The training Marie received from her father, the ballet master and choreographer Filippo Taglioni, prepared her to embody a new romantic style of ballet. He synthesized a style that deemphasized his daughter's overly long arms and neck, her less than beautiful facial features, and the slight hunching forward of her shoulders. Instead, Filippo's training helped to elicit Marie's "airy lightness," her *ballon* (elevation) and soft *ports de bras* (movement of the arms) and the mysteries of her ephemeral balances *sur les pointes.* Filippo and Marie Taglioni extended the balance and the range of movement that could be accomplished while standing on the tips of the toes, the father thus sculpting and crafting an appearance of delicacy and fragile evanescence from his daughter's body.

Such was the popularity of Marie Taglioni's sylphlike image that it was not long before all leading female dancers (especially those like Dumilâtre who were particularly given to the "ethereal" school) adopted softer and more flowing movements of the arms; provocative, even fey inclinations of the head; airy jumps; and deft use of the pointes. Dancers like Dumilâtre, who had achieved some recognition, paid the highest prices to study with masters like Coralli and Filippo Taglioni while those women who remained in the corps de ballet were accommodated in the less costly ballet classes, where they continued to flounder without making substantive progress.[27] For Dumilâtre, though, the acquisition of technique was of primary importance, and she worked to match her increase in strength with a sense of ease and a fluid execution of movement. Significant features of her study were an emphasis on turning out the leg from the hip and top of the thigh, and rising, balancing, and supporting herself on the tips of her toes. She would have learned to dance this way—moving softly onto her full *relevé*—in stiffened slippers that may have been darned on the ends and the sides, but lacked the firm blocking used in the manufacture of the typical pointe shoe of today.

A more extensive use of pointe work for stylistic purposes is one defining characteristic of the ballet technique of the Romantic era. Although the trick of perching on the tips of the toes had long been part of male acrobatic movement vocabularies and had been adopted by numbers of female dancers throughout the early decades of the nineteenth century, it was not until the

1830s that ballet masters began to explore more fully the possibilities of the female dancer's use of the full pointe and her ability to achieve a desirable image of lightness.[28] Paradoxically, to achieve apparent weightlessness required a rigorous and more outwardly extended line of energy and effort through the muscles and limbs. As pointe work became absorbed into the ballerina's arsenal of requisite movement, training methods adapted to accommodate the innovation, incorporating into the classroom exercises a greater emphasis on strengthening the instep, calf, and thigh and support through the pelvis, hips, and abdomen.

Dancing masters of the nineteenth century continued their eighteenth-century predecessors' tradition of publishing dance manuals. Bournonville's legacy—his aesthetics, training philosophies, and choreographies—has been particularly well maintained and documented thanks to the work of the Royal Danish Ballet and research by contemporary scholars.[29] This legacy helps to illuminate the teaching methodologies of masters from the Paris Opéra as Bournonville himself incorporated and revered many of these training practices. In his *A New Year's Gift for Dance Lovers or A View of the Dance as Fine Art and Pleasant Pastime,* written in 1828, Bournonville concentrated on the expressive requirements of the ballet, opening his discussion with the rhetorical question, "Is the dance a fine art?" In his effort to elevate the status of dance as an art form he noted that not only is ballet an activity that causes enjoyment, but the memory of it evokes a "sincere consciousness of the true, the beautiful."[30]

In 1846 when Bournonville, now situated in his native Copenhagen, sent his fifteen-year-old daughter, Augusta, to Paris to study with the great French dancing master Joseph Mazilier, he reminded her to "turn out in all positions, animate your face during exertions, take courage during difficulties and criticism. Be gentle in all your movements. Shun exaggeration and affectation." Beauty, he reminded her, is the goal, and should be the ultimate goal in all training. He encouraged her to practice her turns—he acknowledged that he had difficulty with pirouettes—and always to be careful to stretch her feet. He gave similar advice to his twenty-two-year-old male pupil Johan Ferdinand Hoppe before the latter left for a study tour in Europe. Remember, Bournonville told his student, to guard against "affectation, angular knees, round shoulders, harsh arm movement." Sharpen your memory and your ear, he counseled, and "continually concern yourself with mime, preserve the good school and adopt the beautiful rather than the difficult."[31] The debate underlying Baccelli's training was here echoed by Bournonville: would one sacrifice grace, refinement, and beauty for virtuosity? Though some might call him old school, Bournonville wrote, he proudly acknowledged his confidence in the training he had received from Auguste Vestris, which encouraged the development of virtuosity while retaining the appearance of ease and elegant grace. Bournonville advised another pupil, Jacob Daniel Krum:

> It may be that some call it old fashioned, but novelty which can occur in art is one thing, quite another is that foundation which the beautiful must be built upon and can in no manner be subdued. Therefore, dear friend, grasp whatever can facilitate your genre, assert yourself to win more suppleness in both back and knees, but beware of the style of the circus artist, which is the hallmark of the Italian and French dancers. And above all retain your beautiful entrechat which must be crossed from the hip and not at the foot with disastrous crooked knees which makes the dancer look like a jumping jack.[32]

For Bournonville, the mechanical aspect of dancing was necessary only insofar as it increased the dancer's ability to communicate, but technique was never an end in itself. In *A New Year's Gift* he wrote, "The dancers' preparations may seem as ridiculous as the musicians' scales are boring, yet the result is that, without revealing the work involved, he can create those paintings in movement which a pure imagination can produce." The mastery of technique thus frees the artist to communicate directly to the "soul" of his beholder. Purity, the soul, good taste, and the imagination—these elements, for Bournonville, constitute the "chief aim of art; whosoever achieves [them], is an artist."[33]

Like Bournonville, Gautier championed the creation of beauty. But for Gautier, beauty was an end in itself and he pointedly detached discussions of art from the moral grounding advocated by Bournonville and, earlier, by Noverre. In 1843, Gautier described the romantic revolution as having done away with the "dead" theater of Corneille, Racine, and Molière, the "dead" theater, that is, of Enlightenment rationality and morality. Foreign literature (mainly from Germany and Britain), declared Gautier, had impressed French artists with its imaginative and emotional power. Dramatists turned their backs on mythological themes and embraced depictions of human narratives and human feelings, besides portraying the exotic, the fantastic, and the faraway. The theatrical revolution, claimed Gautier, had broken the yoke of the three unities heretofore conventionally imposed on drama.[34]

Gautier was a man of his time, though, and his well-known pronouncements echoed those of Jules Janin, who, the dance historian John Chapman points out, anticipated his better-known colleague's aesthetic of "*l'art pour l'art*" by at least three years. Janin disparaged the neoclassical "obsession with narrative logic and coherent dramatic action," adding that "logic is a fine thing, but too much logic is intolerable. . . . Why deprive ballet of its most wonderful privileges: disorder, dream, and the absence of common sense?" Like Gautier, Janin advocated an artistic revolution: ballet, he said, is about dance and dancers; it is a divertissement, a thing of beauty and not of ideas. Janin wrote that the ballet "has the great advantage of not being melodrama, tragedy, comedy." Rationality was out of date, proclaimed both Janin and Gautier; reason was the legacy of a too-cerebral emphasis on rules and convention.[35]

Jean-Jacques Rousseau, an early proponent of romanticism, may have helped to initiate the crumbling of the Age of Reason with his publication in 1761 of the "original romantic novel," *La nouvelle Héloïse*. Rousseau's novel had tremendous popular appeal, affecting fashions and changing the way people viewed their world and lived their lives. As many readers understood it, the novel's message could be boiled down to the liberation of the imagination from oppressive rationality. This theme appeared to validate the expression of human feelings and, at root, to indicate that the human heart was fundamentally good.[36] Stirrings of French romanticism were aroused too in response to the defeat of Napoleon at Waterloo in 1815. Many artists sought to counter the authoritarianism and ostentation of Napoleon's reign after his defeat, rejecting the symbols of neoclassicism with which the emperor had chosen to bolster his imperial authority.

Janin and Gautier espoused non-utilitarian art, celebrating beauty for the sake of beauty and beautiful women as works of art. In the 1854 preface to his novel *Mademoiselle de Maupin*, Gautier, delighting in his own irony, wrote, "One of the most ridiculous things in the glorious epoch which we have the happiness to live in is undoubtedly the rehabilitation of virtue."[37] Mocking "modesty" and "virtue," and spurning bourgeois tendencies toward moral and aesthetic complacency, Gautier declared, "Nothing is really beautiful unless it is useless; everything useful is ugly, for it expresses a need, and the needs of man are ignoble and disgusting, like his poor weak nature. The most useful place in a house is the lavatory." And he wrote further, "I should most joyfully renounce my rights as a Frenchman and as a citizen to see an authentic picture by Raphael, or a beautiful woman naked."[38]

Even the bourgeois men and women of ordinary lives and boring "virtue," however, tapped into the new "revolutionary" artistic spirit for, as a cultural mood, romanticism was neither elitist nor obscure. It was, in fact, a movement that infiltrated the lives of everyday women and men. Newly afforded opportunities for universal education, a middle-class French reading public eagerly consumed the otherworldly tales and enticing historical dramas of foreign writers such as Johann Wolfgang Goethe and Walter Scott. Bourgeois men and women applauded the romantic narratives (often in the form of gothic tales) performed nightly on stage at the Paris Opéra. Maurice Cranston explains that the most successful operas between 1826 and 1836, such as Meyerbeer's *Robert le diable* and *Les Huguenots*, Rossini's *Guillaume Tell* and *Moïse*, and Auber's *Gustave III* and *La muette de Portici*, were "costume dramas about sensational clashes of passion in history, and their popularity with Paris audiences signaled the wholehearted acceptance of romanticism by middle-class taste, or at least the acceptance of romanticism in its middlebrow forms."[39] Given such widespread approbation within many levels of society, the romantic artists in the period of about 1815 to 1850 exercised great power over the fashions, tastes, and mores of their times.

The romantic ballet in any of its multiple less-prestigious venues—the Théâtre du Vaudeville, the Cirque Olympique, the Théâtre de la Porte de Ste. Martin, the Théâtre de la Gaîté, the Théâtre du Gymnase Dramatique, or the Théâtre des Variétés, to name just a few places where dance was featured as part of the entertainment—was a world of gaslight, illusion, and beautiful women. It was not, however, an art that was alleged to be terribly serious or profound; while it catered to a bourgeois audience craving beauty and escapist entertainment, most critics and patrons believed it incapable of depicting serious themes or great tragic narratives.

These colorful spectacles were also eagerly consumed by French audiences at the Opéra, where the operating economic structure had been radically altered since the eighteenth century. After the revolutionary struggles of 1830, the overthrow of Charles X, and the institution of a new constitutional monarchy under Louis Philippe ("the Bourgeois King"), the Opéra no longer operated as an arm of an absolutist government. The new director, Dr. Louis Véron, was a private citizen and entrepreneur, answerable to the state but not an appointee of the court. An impresario with his eye trained first and foremost on the balance sheet, Véron was determined to make the Opéra a commercially successful venture, and he invested in a variety of technological innovations. Though the Opéra had been notoriously slow about accepting such change, the boulevard theaters had long made use of a variety of techniques that could heighten theatrical effects and transform the stage into a place of fantasy and illusion.[40] Such stage devices enhanced the popular appeal and commercial viability of the ballets and operas created in the early nineteenth century. Véron's decision to introduce gas lighting, for instance, altered the environment of the Opéra stage, and the use of flying machines allowed for the creation of works borrowing from gothic supernaturalism and the melodrama.[41] Composers assisted in the narration of events by filling their scores with leitmotifs that helped to

45

identify characters and highlight action as the plots unfolded. Printed libretti commonly sold in the foyer prior to the performance also helped clarify the plot, even including lines of dialogue that were never spoken or sung on stage.[42]

Acknowledging audiences who sought diversion and visual spectacle and who generally lacked the classical educations of eighteenth-century audiences, Véron tried hard to give his customers what they wanted. In his memoirs, Véron claimed:

> Dramas and morality plays do not belong in the domain of choreography. Above all, the public demands that a ballet have a striking and varied score, new and unusual costumes, contrasting and novel sets, and a simple, easily understood plot, but one in which the dance develops naturally out of the dramatic situations. One must add to all this the seductiveness of a beautiful young artist, who dances differently from, and more successfully than, those who preceded her. When one speaks neither to the mind nor to the heart, one must speak to the senses, and above all to the eyes.[43]

Ballet's mass appeal was undeniable. The widespread availability of lithographs greatly helped to stir popular interest in ballet and ballerinas by giving audiences access to prints and souvenir albums featuring portraits of their favorite dancers. The ballet girl also became a recurrent figure in favorite literary works of the day. As a sign of their hedonism, the young male roués in the novels of William Thackeray frequently display prints of opera dancers (along with pictures of horses, sporting events, and hunting scenes) on the walls of their apartments. The 1840 sketch entitled "An Invasion of France" depicts chaotic families and gadabout young men who cross the English Channel to visit France. Among Thackeray's travelers is one quite distinct passenger, a French *danseuse* returning to her engagement at the Paris Opéra. Despite its humorous, almost acerbic tone, Thackeray's sharply drawn caricature reveals something of the popular lore about the frivolous flirtatiousness of French ballet dancers: "A *danseuse* from the opera is on her way to Paris. Followed by her *bonne* and her little dog, she paces the deck, stepping out, in the real dancer fashion, and ogling all around. How happy the two young Englishmen are, who can speak French, and make up to her: and how all criticise her points and paces."[44]

Thackeray's caricature points to the economic reality underpinning the livelihood of the French *danseuse:* she flirts with men and they critique her points and paces, associating her with a certain class of men who gambled on horses and ran hunting dogs. Just as they laid wagers on horses, so members of

46

this sporting set often subsidized their favorite *danseuses,* an economic reality that Dr. Véron understood well. Ever attuned to the interests of his male subscribers, Véron opened the *Foyer de la danse* to wealthy men who held season tickets. They were granted access to this mirror-lined rehearsal room where the *danseuses* could be seen completing their warmups and running final rehearsals before stepping out on stage. Véron succeeded in showcasing the foyer as a popular gathering place and in making it fashionable for wealthy scions to "keep" a ballet girl.[45]

Opéra hierarchy dictated that Dumilâtre, like other high-ranking *danseuses,* had private quarters in which to complete her warmup and meet her lovers. Performers who did make use of the foyer, though, usually included members of the *corps de ballet,* or *figurantes* or *marcheuses* who did little beyond walking and posing in groups on stage. Theirs was a different reality. They frequently had very little training and often bore their mothers' names, as their fathers frequently were absent or unknown. Few of these ballet girls genuinely wanted to dance; they were usually placed in the Opéra school by their mothers, who welcomed the few francs their daughters were paid to walk, pose, or dance a little during performances. The poverty and the promiscuity of these lesser dancers almost inevitably led them to lives of prostitution, and it was little surprise that many of them had no dreams beyond one day acquiring their own rich protectors. The truth of such economic hardship was acknowledged by Véron and subsequent directors, and the dancers' desperation was used to increase the Opéra's profit margins.

One view of the seedier side of the French dance world during Dumilâtre's era comes from the journalist Albéric Second. In his book *Les petits mystères de l'Opéra,* Second describes backstage life at the Paris Opéra with a jaunty air. But Second's tongue-in-cheek depiction of the desperate poverty and living conditions of the average young ballet girl at the Paris Opéra (known as a *rat*) lacks the ironic nonchalance of some of his other portraits. The typical story of the young *rat* traced the tortuous progression from desperate poverty and near starvation to the anonymity of the lowest rung of the *corps de ballet.* Second's confidante gives a melodramatic account of girls sent to ballet classes by impoverished mothers, of cold mornings, empty stomachs, and diabolical dancing masters. The confidante also gives insight into the use of painful instruments designed to construct sylphs out of the flesh, bone, and muscle of young women:

> When I was scarcely seven years old, I was sent, to the class of M. Barrez, rue Richer, no. 4. I would leave in the mornings my stomach barely filled by a

weak cup of coffee. I had neither socks nor shoes, nor a shawl for my shoulders, and frequently my poor cotton dress was pierced by the cold as if it were sheer lace. I would arrive shivering and often starving. . . . Each morning, the dancing master would imprison my feet in a grooved box. There, heel against heel and knees forced out, my feet were tortured into remaining locked in a parallel line. That is what one calls turn out. After a half hour in the box, he would make me move on to yet another form of torture.[46]

Louise Robin-Challan has studied the social lives of the Paris Opéra's impoverished ballet girls.[47] About one in seven children sent to the school at the Opéra belonged to a family with theatrical origins; the others came from extremely humble origins. Many mothers who deposited their young daughters at the school were themselves illiterate; while they hoped for a promising future for their children, they signed them over to the school leaving not a name but some insignia, such as a cross. These illiterate and frequently hungry parents, Robin-Challan writes, "belonged to the class of bushel and candle makers, publicans, clothes dealers, washerwomen, concierges, ragmen, people scrubbing floors and doing obscure jobs living from one day into the next." Most often, she says, the families lived far from the site of the Opéra, in "dark attics or a porter's lodge."[48]

The school accepted all children between the ages of seven and ten who arrived at its doors. A medical doctor himself, Dr. Véron examined these children every three months. He took it upon himself to single out the pupils most suited to ballet by examining the general health, temperament, body proportions, and ankle and foot formations of each student. He sent home those he deemed too weak or unfit, a fate that "inevitably meant plunging them into the terrible misery of the poorest of the city. Mothers could implore the director as much as they liked, he remained unaffected: 'a sense of humanity made me uncompromising,' he said."[49]

Those who were kept on at the school lived in conditions that were only slightly more humane. After walking to their morning classes, often without having had any breakfast, the lowliest pupils were put through rigorous exercises: "learning *assemblés, jetés, balancés, ronds de jambe, fouettés, cabrioles, pirouettes sur le cou-de pied, saut de basque, pas-de-bourrée* and, to finish, *entrechats à 4, à 6, à 8.*" Since running water still did not exist in Paris, the girls rarely bathed after their sweat-drenched practice sessions. With poor hygiene, scant food, and extreme overwork, the girls' health was predictably precarious.[50]

Complicating their lives still further, the *rats* were required to pay for their own dance classes. Challan finds that often a male "patron" would pay one hundred francs a month in advance for classes for his girl, essentially speculating on her future. Charles Baudelaire, in his essay "The Painter of Modern Life," wrote about the harsh underworld of the ballet girls: "Now for a moment we move to a lowlier theatrical world where the little dancers, frail, slender, hardly more than children, but proud of appearing at last in the blaze of the limelight, are shaking upon their virginal, puny shoulders absurd fancy dresses which belong to no period, and are their joy and their delight."[51]

These pathetic little dancers were in part responsible for sustaining the social ideology of the day. Popular opinion has long held that the nineteenth-century woman was "the embodiment of domesticity," and that it was largely the social structure provided by the "immoral" women of the theater—Adèle and Sophie Dumilâtre and others further down the professional scale—who allowed this notion of the "good" woman to be perpetuated. By the end of the 1790s, according to the social historian James F. McMillan, the French craved a stable social environment, in reaction to what they perceived as the Revolution's disruption of the natural order of gender relationships.[52] But notions of legitimacy and of the "natural" order were upheld and supported by social conventions that dictated a sexual double standard. "Given that bourgeois men were expected to acquire sexual experience while women of their class were required to retain their virginity until marriage, it followed that male debauchery could not take place in the beds of decent, well-brought up young ladies. But if bourgeois men idealised the chastity of their own womenfolk, they regarded other, less fortunate women as fair game."[53] While girls in bourgeois families were sheltered and generally restricted in their opportunities to venture forth into the world, the impoverished ballet girls, as well as the more renowned ballerinas, were often the ones who satisfied the societal demand for sexually available women. In any case, a culture that asked its mothers, daughters, and wives to be "angels" relied on its "fallen" sisters to support and sustain its idealizations.

In his eighth letter in *Letters on Dance and Choreography,* Bournonville addressed the reality he knew to exist backstage at the Paris Opéra. He wrote the following stunning indictment of the conditions of the average young ballet girl:

> Look at that phalanx of sylphs maintaining a carefree smile whilst holding their dying sister in their arms! This light-hearted group consists of two categories of female dancers: the first who hope to achieve talent, and the second who forever will be frustrated by it. The first group consists of the youngest and usually the prettiest. They have been reared in poverty but with a lot of ambition. The only reward for their hard work is, in most cases, the meagre nourishment provided by parents impatient to see them *earn their living!*

They must pay their teacher and *behave themselves*, and the administration employs them *gratis* or for an insignificant fee. The others, older and less gifted by nature, have seen all their efforts frustrated by the twin obstacles of a poor physique and bad luck; they do their duty, cast an indifferent glance at the brilliantly gifted, and try to banish from their thoughts the prospect of retirement, often without any hope of a pension; happy to be able to aspire to a job as an usherette!—They receive an annual salary ranging from one-thousand to four hundred francs! And their dances are meant to portray an image of sensuous enjoyment.—*Cruel irony!*[54]

Cruel irony, indeed, for at the opposite extreme, Véron could also bank on heightened audience excitement about dance and dancers by marketing the competition between his most prominent ballerinas. He created a public stir by inflaming rivalries, such as the one between Fanny Elssler (Gautier's "Pagan" or earthy ballerina) and Marie Taglioni (the "Christian," or "spiritual" dancer). The press played its part in publicizing such rivalries since the dual roles embodied by these two dancers echoed the polarities characterizing romantic aesthetics.

The claque, another institution of tremendous power in the theater, electrified the public all the more and enhanced the public rivalry between ballerinas. The so-called *chef-du-claque* (the most famous of whom was the notorious Auguste Levasseur) determined audience reception to individual dancers. The *chef* wielded this control over the ballet and opera, having been previously bought off by the director or the artists themselves with gifts of free seats. The *chef*, in his turn, operated a network of lieutenants and sublieutenants who weighed heavily in controlling the volume of applause or hisses with which an *artiste* was greeted. Véron describes in his memoirs the evening when he maneuvered a less-than-favorable response to the ballerina Pauline Duvernay because he believed her mother was getting out of hand. When *Maman* began making too many demands on her daughter's behalf, Véron retained the upper hand by arranging for Pauline's solo turn to be greeted with a deadening silence. According to Véron, Madame Duvernay's pride was, for a time, taken down several notches.

On several occasions, Adèle Dumilâtre herself had recourse to outside forces to manipulate her career. In several instances she resorted to the powers of the journalist Charles Maurice. Dumilâtre wrote to him from London on September 29, 1845, for example, to say she had won public favor since she had been greeted with bravos and "we were obliged to start our dance over again." She closed the letter by thanking Maurice in advance for all that he would do for her in his future recommendations of her, and by expressing gratitude for his extreme good-will toward her.[55] Altogether in a different mood, Dumilâtre requested the journalist's aid when she wrote from Milan on January 20, 1846, distraught at having been denied a chance to perform. "I would have written to you sooner if I had not been so greatly distressed," she writes. "The Director has decided to bring in another dancer to dance *Le Diable à Quatre* in my place because the public has made a terrible fuss every evening, demanding the other ballet." And in closing, she names names: "I learned that it was Mademoiselle Andrianoff who is going to come here to take my place. . . . I beg you to continue your kindly support of me."[56]

On the one hand the Opéra was home to ambitious career women like Dumilâtre who wielded some power to improve their situations; on the other hand, however, there were those dancers Baudelaire referred to as the "children" of the lowlier theatrical world. Each of these conflicting impressions of female dancers at the Paris Opéra during the flowering of the romantic ballet bears a truth to life. The multiplicity of such impressions attests to the hierarchical standards as well as the commercialism that dictated the creation of ballets and the allocation of roles; to the bitterness and rivalry that reigned backstage; to the gravity of some women's circumstances; and, paradoxically, to the very glory and rich creativity of the period.

—————

More than a century after its premiere, *Giselle* (1841) was described by the twentieth-century dance critic Cyril Beaumont as "the supreme achievement of the Romantic Ballet," because of its amalgamation of the local color and charm of the first act's peasant world, and the second act's evocation of the ethereal, fantastic wilis.[57] Gautier's essay of June 28, 1841, describes how the French poet came across the German folk tale that inspired the ballet:

> My dear Heinrich Heine, while leafing through your excellent book, *De l'Allemagne*, a few weeks ago, my eyes rested on a charming passage . . . in which you speak of the white-robed elfs whose hems are ever damp, the nixes who display their little satin feet on the ceiling of the nuptial chamber, the pallid wilis and their pitiless waltz, and all those delightful apparitions which you encountered in the Harz mountains and on the banks of the Ilse in the velvety mists of German moonlight—and involuntarily I said to myself, "What a lovely ballet that would make!"[58]

The ballet, according to Gautier, was meant to be as delightful and diverting as the above passage suggests. It should evoke nothing of serious import and should allow audiences seeking an escape from hard reality the opportunity to indulge in beauty for its own sake.

A lithograph published in London in 1843 gives an idealized look at how Dumilâtre appeared to audiences in her role as Myrtha. Here, a full-bosomed Dumilâtre is poised on unnaturally slender legs, balancing on the tip of her right pointe, with her left leg in an arabesque raised hip height to the back. She circles both arms over her head. Her right hand clasps the branch of rosemary that Queen Myrtha uses to summon her entourage. Dumilâtre's head is turned toward the front and though there is no softness in her face, the artist hints at what were popularly considered her most beautiful features: a slender, elegant neck and a shapely, oval face. She is costumed in a gauzy white, multilayered skirt that hangs to midcalf. A cross is visible on her right, along with a shrouded female standing as if awaiting Myrtha's commands. A castle can be seen in the background, off in the distance beyond the forested landscape that encircles the two supernaturals.

In the libretto as it was eventually worked out by the well-known stage librettist Vernoy de Saint-Georges, *Giselle* is the story of a beautiful young peasant girl who is doomed by both her weak heart and her excessive love of dancing.[59] Giselle's mother, Berthe, repeatedly warns that her love for dance will lead Giselle to an early grave and resurrection as a vampire-like wili: a spirit maiden who—in life—loved dancing too much and who, because she was jilted before marriage, is fated—after death—to wreak vengeance on all men who wander into her gloomy forest surroundings at night. In spite of Berthe's persistent fears, Giselle runs away from her chores at every opportunity, choosing instead to dance away the daylight hours. When the passionate but innocent young peasant girl falls in love with a philandering lord named Albrecht (or Albert), who is disguised as a peasant hunter calling himself Loys, she is doomed forever. Hilarion, a coarse but loyal huntsman who is jealous of Giselle's affections, discovers Albrecht's masquerade and reveals his rival's noble status as well as his betrothal to a noblewoman, Bathilde. A confrontation ensues between the two men, and Giselle goes mad, dying of her overstrained emotions and her ailing heart. The ballet's first act closes with a dramatic tableau: Giselle lies dead, her body cradled by her weeping mother, in the center of the stage. Poised around the mother and daughter are Hilarion and Albrecht, distraught and combative, each blaming the other for the beloved girl's death. Grouped around these central characters are Giselle's peasant friends from the village. Their poses, attitudes, and facial expressions depict grief, shock, and despair.

The second act opens in the midnight realm dominated by Myrtha and her legion of wilis. Gautier engages all sensory perceptions in recreating the scene:

The stage represents a forest by the edge of a lake, overhung by tall pale trees with their roots steeped in the grass and the bullrushes, and with water lilies spreading their broad leaves on the placid surface of the water silvered here and there by the moon with a trail of white patches. Reeds emerge from their smooth brown sheaths to shiver and tremble in the intermittent night breeze. The flowers are half open, languidly spreading their heady scent like those large blooms of Java that madden all who inhale them, and a sort of burning sensuous atmosphere circulates in this dense and humid darkness. At the foot of a willow tree, lost and embedded among the flowers, lies Giselle. On the white marble cross that marks her grave hangs, still fresh, the crown of leaves with which she was crowned at the vintage festival.[60]

Jules Janin was a great admirer of the ballet and of the ballerinas who starred in the premiere, Carlotta Grisi as Giselle and Dumilâtre as Myrtha. In his review of June 30, 1841, Janin described Dumilâtre's entrance this way: "The vapor is Myrtha, the Queen of the Wilis. The first rays of the September moon have given Myrtha the fine contours of her beautiful form. A strange light accompanies her mysterious majesty. She has wings because it is her whim, a white tunic because it is the fashion at balls given under old oaks to the song of crickets, beating bat wings, and the thousand unexpected laments murmured in the forest's gloomy depths. Let us begin! Sleepy Wilis, arise! It is your queen who commands you."[61] In Janin's critique, the separation between real-life woman and dangerous supernatural is blurred, and flesh-and-blood ballerinas become merged with their ethereal stage personas. As wilis they are alluring; as women they are dangerously and seductively beautiful. The dangerous creature is not solely a stage role, though. For Janin, Dumilâtre is Myrtha and she is a "temptress": "She is young and beautiful, well made, sweetly blooming, and pretty beyond the usual Opéra prettiness. Bitten by the most innocent of tarantulas, she obeys with joy. Giselle had to be very powerful, indeed, for her lover to resist this elegant Wili of eighteen years."[62]

According to the hierarchy of the wilis' supernatural world, Myrtha/Adèle was assisted by two lieutenants, Zulmé (the *Bayadère*, the Indian wili), danced by Sophie Dumilâtre, and Moyna (the odalisque, the oriental wili), danced by Mademoiselle Carré. In productions even today, when the forlorn huntsman, Hilarion, arrives to mourn at Giselle's cross, he is promptly packed off to his demise by the unrelentingly vengeful wilis. Myrtha then commands that Giselle emerge from her grave so that she may be initiated into the corps of vampire maidens. The newcomer dances on command, but even Myrtha's fierce power cannot force Giselle to forsake her love for Albrecht. When the distraught lover makes his way into the forest at midnight to grieve and place lilies at the grave of his beloved Giselle, he is sure prey for the deadly, vindictive maidens. Demanding that he dance until he die, Myrtha wields a futile command since the eternal love of the two allows Giselle to sustain her mortal lover until he collapses from fatigue just at dawn—exhausted but alive.

In the second act it is made apparent that in spite of his perfidy, Albrecht indeed feels remorse, and that Giselle's love for him is true and abiding. It is eternal love and its redemptive power that is the focus of most contemporary performances of the ballet. Nevertheless, the original libretto included several additional details that have faded from most productions today. One of these features was the distinction of the wilis' various lands of origin (for instance, Zulmé comes from India, and Moyna, from the Orient). Adolphe Adam incorporated representative musical themes into his music to clarify the wilis' various national origins. Though these melodies are mostly indistinguishable to contemporary listeners, Lisa C. Arkin and Marian Smith point out that nineteenth-century audiences would have "recognized the ethnic references in the brief snippets of Spanish and 'Eastern'-sounding music that Adam wove into what he called the 'fantastic ball' scene of Act II, presumably to accompany the foreign Wilis as they executed what Adam called 'the figures of their native dance.'"[63]

Smith and Arkin additionally describe the original extensive mime passages that have gradually been whittled away in response to contemporary audiences' preference for "pure dance" over gesture and narrative. Also, Myrtha and her vengeful spirits at one time received a number of incidental guests to their eerie forest, including a band of hunters who take to their heels after being thoroughly terrified by the ghostly women. And in the distance there would have been a gathering of jovial peasants who wandered astray after too much carousing. In 1841, the wilis gave chase but the festive band of healthy, fun-loving mortals eluded them. The ballet's final redemptive scene, in which Giselle gives her lover over to a future with a living woman, is a gesture that is most noticeably absent today. At the end of act 2, scene 13, in Gautier's libretto, the noble lover's servant, Wilfrid, runs into the moonlit graveyard to save his prince from the wilis. Meanwhile dawn spreads in the sky and the wilis approach their last moments on earth. Albrecht is struck with grief and surprise at seeing Giselle slowly descend into her grave. But, as she begins to vanish from his view, she makes a final gesture toward Bathilde, who is seen kneeling a few steps away from Albrecht, holding out her hand toward him pleadingly. Giselle seems to indicate that her lover should give his love and faith to Bathilde; this is her last wish and her prayer. It is the wish, says Gautier, of one who can no longer love him in this world, a benediction from one whose wishes Albrecht now holds sacred. Giselle then disappears from view as Albrecht rises with a visible sadness, tears up some of the flowers that cover Giselle's grave, and, weak with love and sorrow, presses them to his heart and his lips. As the curtain falls, he can be seen holding the hand of his betrothed, the noblewoman Bathilde.

Ultimately, Janin registered his satisfaction with the *Giselle:* "Nothing is missing from this charming work: there is invention, poetry, music, newly arranged dances, lots of pretty danseuses, lively harmony, grace, energy, Adèle Dumilâtre, and, especially, *la* Carlotta Grisis. This, for sure, is what a ballet should be!"[64]

On June 1, 1840, Léon Pillet was appointed director of the Paris Opéra, replacing Dr. Louis Véron. Along with the directorship, Pillet assumed the obligation to produce a specified number of new ballets and operas each year. In 1844, though, Pillet found himself in a real "quandary," since, as Guest writes, "he could see little prospect of presenting his one star ballerina, Carlotta Grisi, in a new ballet, and after her he was left with three ballerinas of considerably lesser magnitude." These remaining ballerinas included Pauline Leroux and Maria Jacob (the latter usually known onstage only by her first name), each of whom was deemed unfit to undertake the lead in an important new ballet. Pillet's third available ballerina was Adèle Dumilâtre, who was young, beautiful, very ambitious, and outfitted with a number of important protectors. When Saint-Georges submitted his libretto for a new ballet entitled *Lady Henriette ou la servante de Greenwich,* Pillet thought seriously of giving the lead role to Dumilâtre. After further consideration, however, he decided that this was too risky since her youthful talents and as yet limited fame might not support such an expensive work. He was convinced otherwise by the sudden donation of a substantial sum of money by one of Dumilâtre's patrons. Guest explains:

> Hearing of [Pillet's doubts], Edouard Monnais, the Royal Commissioner whose duty it was to supervise the expenditure of the subsidy, summoned Pillet to his office. Pillet explained that he was reluctant to incur the heavy outlay which the new ballet entailed with a dancer of only Dumilâtre's standing in the leading role. Monnais did not insist, but a few days later a gentleman was shown into Pillet's office and offered the sum of 100,000 francs if the ballet were produced for Dumilâtre with all possible speed.[65]

The ballet's plot was not an original one for it had first appeared in *Ballet des chambrières à louer* and would later be seen in the vaudeville performance *La comtesse d'Egmont.*[66] Still, the scenario as produced by Saint-Georges was less than entirely appropriate for the ballet stage, as Gautier chided in his review

55

in *La Presse,* on February 26, 1844. Although the première was a complete success, Gautier charged that Saint-Georges "sometimes overlooks the fact that a ballet should be a picture before being a drama." Instead, said Gautier, "M. de Saint-Georges' work belongs more to the form that is termed *ballet d'action,* or putting it in another way, in which dancing occupies only a secondary place."[67] Although nothing of the choreography of *Lady Henriette* survives today, the production suggests a somewhat hodge-podge affair. In order to expedite the ballet's première, three composers, Burgmuller, Develdez, and Flotow, were each commissioned to compose music for one of three acts.[68] With choreography by Mazilier and sets by Cicéri, the ballet was first performed at the Opéra on February 21, 1844.

Set in England, "not one of the most choreographic of countries," Gautier alleges, the ballet-pantomime takes place in the eighteenth-century court of Queen Anne. Lady Henriette/Dumilâtre is a frivolous and bored lady-in-waiting to the queen. Gautier retells the story by including lines of dialogue that could only have been mimed on stage. The charming Lady Henriette has become indifferent to her life: finery and jewelry no longer divert her, music no longer interests her, and she is irritated by her husband-to-be, the "pretentious imbecile" Sir Tristan Crakford, who is, says Gautier, "the most unbearable fool imaginable." As the ballet opens, Lady Henriette is engaged in tormenting her betrothed—"Pick up my handkerchief," "Fetch my fan," "Open the window," "Close it"—but even this game begins to wear on her overstrained nerves. Gautier's description of what happens next resembles the narration of a play: "The sound of a rustic march is heard. 'What is that, Nancy?' Lady Henriette asks her faithful companion, who is leaning over the balcony. 'Young girls who are unemployed, coming to the servants' fair to look for a master and a situation.'" Lady Henriette bids the female rustics to enter her room, and she is, continues Gautier, "suddenly struck by a crazy idea. The short skirt, little cap and straw bouquet [which the village girls carry] would suit her to perfection, and she has the sudden whim to dress up as a young village girl and, accompanied by her companion Nancy, go and look for a situation in the servants' fair."[69] Costume plates from the Maison Martinet, Hautecoeur Frères, in Paris show that Adèle, costumed as a servant girl, wore a full skirt reaching to midcalf, a blouse with sleeves that ballooned out above her elbows, a peasant bodice, and a Bretonne cap on her head.[70]

At the fair, the young farmer, Lyonnel, danced by Lucien Petipa, is struck by Henriette's beauty and hires her as a servant. Nancy is hired by his comrade, "a short, fat, thick-set farmer with a complexion like a nut, a friend of Lyonnel by the name of Plunkett."[71] Carrying their ruse forward, Lady Henriette and her maid accompany their new employers home, but they rebel upon being asked to do household chores. In spite of the rebellious nature of his "serving girl," Lyonnel finds that he has fallen in love with her. Suddenly Lady Henriette begins to realize the potential gravity of her playful masquerade, and she and Nancy take the first opportunity to escape that night. The women return to their lives in Queen Anne's court and Henriette is once again plagued by the attentions of her betrothed, Sir Crakford.

The next act takes viewers to the royal forest at Windsor, where the hunting party of Queen Anne overtakes a group of soldiers. Audiences would have seen Adèle in her hunting outfit, a full, floor-length skirt and a riding jacket with broad cuffs, a blouse, a sash, and a scarf or bow at the neck. A noble woman's flat hunting hat with a slightly upturned brim was perched on her head. As might be expected, Lyonnel recognizes his beloved as she lies resting apart from the others in the hunting party. He approaches her only to be spurned. He is about to leave the scene in despair over the unkindness of the woman he loves when suddenly the queen's horse bolts out of control. He darts forward to grasp the reins of the wildly galloping horse, thus saving the life of the queen. In her gratitude the queen presents him with a ring, which, she tells him, he can present to her in the future to be granted any wish he desires. Then she appoints him one of her guards. Lady Henriette, in the meanwhile, has disappeared from the forest.

The next scene transports the audience to the interior of Windsor Castle, where preparations are underway for the presentation of a mythological divertissement. The queen takes the part of Juno while the role of Venus goes to Lady Henriette, who, Gautier records, "performs it scrupulously well at least from point of view of beauty, for she shows a Hyrcanian cruelty towards poor Lyonnel, who recognising her when he comes to change guard, loses his head to such an extent that he becomes mad with rage and sorrow and has to be incarcerated in Bedlam, where we find him in the following scene."[72]

The ballet then enters Bedlam, where the benevolent Queen Anne and her ladies have gone to visit the infirm lunatics. Once again, Henriette is confronted by Lyonnel, who has by now been rendered mad through his disappointed love for her. "The sight of him melts [Henriette's] proud ice-cold heart, and she confesses to the queen how her thoughtlessness has had such dreadful consequences, and that all she wants to do now is to make amends." The ballet ends happily as the formerly disdainful Lady Henriette learns to love her once rejected Lyonnel. And with the presentation of his ring to the queen, Lyonnel is of course granted the hand of the lady he has pursued and whose coldness has only temporarily caused him to go mad.[73]

In concluding his review, Gautier described Mademoiselle Adèle Dumilâtre in her role as Lady Henriette:

> It was the first time that this beautiful dancer had created a leading rôle in an important work, and she came through the difficult ordeal with flying colours. She has a remarkable elegance and distinction, and in her village costumes revealed a charming coquetry and affected artlessness that well befitted a Countess pretending to be a servant. As for her dances, which consist of a *pas de demi-caractère* with Petipa in the first act and a *pas de Vénus* with Henri Desplaces in the second, she was applauded on several occasions, particularly in the mythological *pas*, which she rendered with the nobility of attitude, the aerial lightness and the modest grace that are her particular qualities. There can be no purer profile, nor a more limpid, bluer glance. One of our dreams is to see Mlle. Dumilâtre play one of those pale divinities who appear in Northern legends. What a pretty elf she would make in the Harz mountains, and what an admirable Valkyrie in Odin's Valhalla! All of which does not prevent her from being a charming English Countess in M. de Saint-Georges' ballet.[74]

The role clearly allowed Dumilâtre to engage in some lively character acting and the sort of light-hearted stage play that moved her beyond the regal and frosty demeanor of Myrtha, queen of the wilis. From a dramatic standpoint, she made the transition from an aristocrat with a "proud ice-cold heart" to a loving and humbled woman, willing to accept Lyonnel's devotion and take him for her husband. But the ballet, with its pastiche of scores (Gautier ranked the Burgmüller score as being the superior), has not endured. Sophie Dumilâtre danced the role of Mina, Lyonnel's rejected fiancée, but Adèle and her Lyonnel, Lucien Petipa, carried the day.

THE DUMILÂTRE LEGACY

In a lithograph depicting a lively partnering pose from *The Corsair*, Henri Desplaces supports Dumilâtre, holding her out to his side.[75] She appears to be floating aloft, her legs extending behind, as if Desplaces has caught her around the waist midjump, at the height of a *cabriole* or a *brisé*. The partnering stance is improbable as Desplaces is not entirely stable—he has one leg extended in a *tendu* back, and he appears to support her without effort. The stance suggests that she is weightless and that he restrains her from floating away. Both dancers look out at the viewer; Desplaces glances over his right shoulder, while Dumilâtre faces front, her arms circling her head, her long braids swinging behind her back. He wears a short tunic that is belted at the waist and reaches to midthigh. She is dressed in a layered skirt with brocaded bodice; a pert

"Turkish" cap perches on the back of her head. The lithograph emphasizes Dumilâtre's slender oval face, her long neck, and her airy lightness.

As a woman who showed an early talent, Dumilâtre probably saw little of the world outside the ballet studio and the stage prior to her retirement in 1848. She may have been a cosseted prodigy, given, as Edward Binney puts it, her "almost-unique distinction of having 'a ballet father.'"[76] That she was ambitious seems likely, for she faced formidable challenges from noted ballerinas such as Taglioni, Elssler, and Grisi. Dumilâtre was more than simply an average talent, and her career was more than modest. Judging from the evidence, it seems natural to assume that she worked diligently to grow as an artist and to fulfill her professional goals. I do not suppose she took her talent for granted; indeed, a surviving letter dated only "Londres 29 Septembre" suggests otherwise. The letter, written in French, is simply addressed to "Monsieur"; in the body of the letter, Dumilâtre congratulates the choreographer of *La fille de marbre* on the success he has had at the première performance of his work. The newspapers, she writes, are unanimous in confirming this brilliant success, and she expresses gratitude for having been chosen for the role. She states that she will redouble her efforts to deserve the honor of being chosen the interpreter of this role.[77]

Restrained qualities of elegance and delicacy are suggested in a portrait of Dumilâtre by Léon Noël, after Joseph Negelen (Paris, 1843).[78] Looking distinctly unlike a courtesan in this portrait, Dumilâtre stands quietly, dressed in a gown with modest neckline and short, capped sleeves. In a gesture of poise and serenity, she rests one hand on the low wall behind her; a single bracelet graces her long, elegant forearm. Her waist is encircled by a sash, and her shawl, which drapes around her arms, hangs low around her hips. Her delicate oval face is framed by tightly bound, sleek black hair that is parted in the middle, swept across her ears, and gathered behind her head. Her eyes are large, her eyelashes modestly lowered; her nose is long and slender. She is a picture of easy, untroubled grace.

In what ways is Dumilâtre's presence felt today? Is something of her dancing preserved in the skimming *pas de bourrées* of our present-day Myrthas? Is she somehow embodied in the "womanly Myrtha" of Carmen Corella, or in the "majestic" presence of Michele Wiles?[79] Is she there in the light and yet "grand" movement quality of Martine Van Hamel?[80] Does she linger in the steps, body, and characterization of Maria Alexandrova, "a statuesque dancer in the grand, expressive Bolshoi style," whose evocation of the role is "stern but exciting"?[81] I am certain that traces of her artistry live on in all of these contemporary interpretations.

3
TAMARA
KARSAVINA

TAMARA KARSAVINA'S well-known and well-loved memoir, *Theatre Street,* reveals what went on within the legendary Imperial Theatre School in St. Petersburg, Russia, during the final years of the nineteenth century. There, mythic dancers like Anna Pavlova and Vaslav Nijinsky were trained and coached in the performance of ballets choreographed by the great ballet master Marius Petipa. Karsavina's reminiscences helped to open doors to the transplantation of ballet from Europe to Russia, and the subsequent emergence of the Diaghilev Ballets Russes, which reintroduced classical ballet to many twentieth-century audiences in western Europe and America. Karsavina's book puts in perspective her connections to other legendary figures of the period, among them Fokine, Nijinska, Rubinstein, Bakst, Rambert, Stravinsky, Balanchine, and Massine. A ballerina at the Maryinsky Ballet and the primary female interpreter of Michel Fokine's choreography, Karsavina achieved status in the history of ballet that is unchallenged. Yet the intelligence, independence, courage, and resilience that Karsavina sustained throughout her life are not widely recognized, as she typically has been portrayed as just one of the many satellites circling Sergei Diaghilev. In fact, she was one of the most renowned dancers of the early twentieth century. Quietly and without drawing undue attention to herself, she was also a model of female strength and self-reliance. Karsavina married for love, escaped from revolutionary Russia, raised a child, and spoke and wrote in three languages. She was the main breadwinner for her family for a number of years; she taught, coached, wrote about her experiences and about ballet technique, and never lost her vibrant interest in life.

One account of her life is given in her memoirs, but a different picture—of the sometimes demure and reticent but often vivacious woman—emerges in *Thirty Dozen Moons,* the story told by her second husband, the English diplomat H. J. (Benjie) Bruce. She figures too as the pixieish, fun-loving friend to the dancer Lydia Kyasht, who, in her *Romantic Recollections,* recalls their games, pranks, and first loves while the two were students at the Imperial Ballet School.[1] Karsavina also makes her appearance, in some fashion, in numerous other accounts, ranging from Michel Fokine's *Memoirs of a Ballet Master* to Peter Lieven's *The Birth of the Ballets-Russes,* and including Arnold Haskell's and Cyril Beaumont's extensive writings on the Diaghilev Ballet, Richard Buckle's biographies of Diaghilev and Nijinsky, and Buckle's *In the Wake of Diaghilev.* She crops up in Margot Fonteyn's *Autobiography* as the *grande dame* who coached the English ballerina in ballets such as *Le spectre de la rose, Firebird,* and *Giselle,* and her presence is evoked in books about Ninette de Valois and Frederick Ashton. She appears as a silent, dancing character in a whimsically eccentric play called *The Truth about Russian Dancers,* by Sir James M. Barrie, the Scottish author.[2] More recently Karsavina has figured prominently in books and articles by Lynn Garafola (especially her *Diaghilev's Ballets Russes*) and in Sally Banes's *Dancing Women.*

However, there is far more to her story than is typically conveyed in the numerous historical accounts of the Diaghilev Ballets Russes, where she figures as a beloved ballerina and a marketable commodity in Diaghilev's enterprise. Less well known is her vast contribution to the development of ballet in Britain, where she was a mentor to the young English choreographer Frederick Ashton and advised the establishment of the Association of Teachers of Operatic Dancing (later the Royal Academy of Dancing) in the United Kingdom.

Karsavina's female strength is also underappreciated. One could guess that she was passionate about her dancing and that she would be disciplined, focused, and strong in pursuing her career. But she was equally passionate about her family life and often felt torn between her obligations to her career and her private time with her loved ones. She possessed a toughness that enabled her to make the transition from an aristocratic society based on an Old World model to an entirely different culture in western Europe. She had a kind of fortitude that allowed her to support Fokine in his decision to rebel politically as well as artistically. Her intellectual curiosity aligned her with Diaghilev and his avant-garde artistic circles.

Tamara Platonovna Karsavina was born March 9, 1885, in St. Petersburg, Russia, and died May 26, 1978, in Beaconsfield, England. The account
of Karsavina's relocation from her country of birth to England, where she
resided for many years with her British husband and their son, encompasses
her personal artistic journey, traces the spread of ballet in western Europe,
and highlights the great decades during which she danced with the legendary
Diaghilev Ballets Russes. It was the British balletomane and critic Arnold
Haskell who encouraged Karsavina to write her memoir, which she did in
English, and which resulted in the publication of *Theatre Street* in 1930.[3] Her
recollections of her training at the famed Imperial Theatre School helped to
convince British audiences of the legitimate place of the ballet among the
artistic and cultural elite in Russia. Readers of her memoir discovered that,
unlike the lowly, uneducated western European "ballet girls," Russian dancers graduated from a disciplined and convent-like institution where matrons
maintained strict separations between boy and girl students and sheltered
young dancers from the outside world. The school drew its students from
socially respectable circles and, as befitted servants of the tsar, they were well-
educated and highly trained artists.[4]

Karsavina depicts her family life prior to her school years, when she lived
with her father, a "first dancer and mime at the Imperial Ballet"; her stern but
"rational" mother; and her brilliant brother, Lev. She speaks of her precocious
love of reading, which was unchecked by her parents, who let her read through
the volumes of Pushkin that her father kept on his bookshelves: "Such is the
divine simplicity of Poushkin's verse," she writes, "and such the limpidity of
his prose that even to me, a child of six, it set no riddles; and, though unable
to analyse the beauty of his writing, I felt it by instinct. His magic spell has
never since loosened its grasp on me."[5] Her roving intellect and her passionate
responses to art and literature were to bolster her life and career.

Her father, Platon Konstaninovich Karsavin, was the methodical, careful,
first teacher of the young Michel Fokine.[6] Platon Karsavin had once been
a favorite pupil of the great French ballet master Marius Petipa, but something—Karsavina says she did not know what it was—soured their relations.
When her memoir opens, her father faces a premature retirement from the
stage owing to this unspecified political intrigue:

> Mother always had a high courage. Nothing ever daunted her, and now she
> hoped that, with more time on his hands, Father would be able to get more
> lessons, and that things would be all right. But I think the blow to their pride

meant more than financial considerations to them. After all, we always lived from hand to mouth, never looking ahead, spending more when there was something to spend, fitting in somehow when there wasn't. Father had reason to expect his being kept for the second service, like other artists of his standing. He was sore at heart parting with the stage.[7]

Though Karsavin continued as a teacher at the Imperial Theatre School and retained some private pupils, the frustration and disappointment of this early retirement led him to forbid his daughter to study ballet, but Karsavina's strong-willed mother disagreed. While she had never considered the ballet an appropriate career for a man, "Mother's dream was to make a dancer of me," Karsavina writes. "'It is a beautiful career for a woman,' she would say, 'and I think the child must have a leaning for the stage; she is fond of dressing up, and always at the mirror.'"[8] Lev, she said, must have a superior education, but the schooling at the Imperial Ballet School was absolutely appropriate for Tamara. Even if she never became a "great" dancer, her mother reasoned, her salary as a dancer in the *corps de ballet* would be greater than any other wage available to an educated woman in tsarist Russia. Since the girl was excluded from the highest university education because of her gender, the mother believed that Tamara should have some socially acceptable means of supporting herself. Ironically, in spite of such exclusion, Karsavina's own native intellect and passion for reading and art would eventually win her renown as one of the most intelligent and intellectually advanced ballerinas of her era.

According to Karsavina, the decision to dance was one she would have made for herself, for she harbored the notion of being on the stage long before she was taken to the theater for the first time. Her father, however, did not want to subject his daughter to the "intrigues of the stage." Further, he predicted, "she will be like me, too meek to stand up for herself."[9] Ignoring his resistance, Karsavina's mother secretly started the young girl in lessons with a family friend, Madame Joukova, a retired dancer.

Though Karsavina dreamed of leaping and turning right away, her ballet training was conducted in the "orthodox" Russian manner. As Karsavina recalled Joukova's methodology, "For the first two months she kept me to bar practice; and only when my feet were turned out properly did she begin to give me some exercises in the centre." The process was one of "gradual and systematic practice" that was "spread over seven or eight years. Before the end of that period no dancer is considered for the stage."[10] Karsavina's mother finally approached Platon Karsavin with the news that their daughter had been taking ballet lessons for months. Apparently his rebukes were mild as he simply pointed out that Tamara would be the third generation of the Karsavin family on the stage. Karsavina then began taking lessons with her father. A normally gentle-natured man, her father was a "most exacting teacher, and when he sat there, his ever-present glass of tea by his side, he even assumed some sternness of manner. To the tune of his fiddle I exerted myself to the utmost. He never considered I had done my best unless sweat trickled down my face. He told me that when he worked for his début he literally sweated blood." He peppered her with "sharp, pithy remarks," such as, "do not hold your arms like candelabras; knees bent like an old horse," and sometimes he "swished" her legs with his fiddlesticks. Karsavina writes that her father belonged "to the old school of masters who believed that, unless a rigorous discipline is established, the pupil will let himself go."[11]

Her audition for the Imperial Theatre School was etched in Karsavina's memory, as the young students were duly marched into a vast chamber to be examined by ballet teachers as well as by physicians. They were then tested in reading, writing, math, and musical scales. A formidable and austere event under the best of conditions, the process was even more intimidating for Karsavina, for although her father was on the examination panel, he refused to return her gaze or notice her in any special way. Over thirty children were called upon to walk, then run, and then stand with their heels together. After this examination, some were dismissed as physically unsuited to the training. Those who remained were sent to the infirmary for thorough medical examinations. At the end of the day, she was one of the ten students selected for the school, and, she recalled, she passed a rather uneventful first year with uninspiring teachers.

The Imperial Ballet school preserved an autocratic way of life that excluded any breath of the revolutionary ferment seething, and occasionally erupting, outside its walls during the late nineteenth and early twentieth centuries. "The fashion of our clothes belonged to the preceding century, but was well in keeping with the spirit of the institution, with its severe detachment from the life outside its walls," Karsavina writes. "Vowed to the theatre, we were kept from contact with the world as from a contamination."[12] The life of the theater, its stars, and its intrigues became all-consuming. The young dancers separated themselves into two camps, avidly declaring their allegiance either to the principal ballerina, Mathilde Kschessinska, or to her rival ballerina, Olga Preobrajenskaya. They were also to declare their "adoration" for one of their masters. Karsavina's choice was Pavel Gerdt. "Though over forty, he ever remained the 'first lover' on the stage, and his looks did not betray him."[13]

Accepted stage policy dictated that Gerdt, though all but retired from active dancing because of knee injuries, still partnered the ballerina as the *danseur noble*, the handsome lover, in the *grand pas de deux*, while the more active male dancing role would be given over to a younger dancer. "Fair and handsome, he was almost boyish on the stage, a first-rate actor," Karsavina writes about Gerdt. Her adoration was well placed; Gerdt was also her godfather and frequently visited her family at home, always bringing her a large box of chocolates. At the time of her schoolgirl "adoration," she could not foresee that at her milestone debut in 1907 as Medora in *Le corsaire*, it would be Gerdt who would partner her in the role of her beloved, Conrad.

Gerdt proved to be her most influential teacher. According to Natalia Roslavleva, it was the soft movement flow and beautiful use of the arms that distinguished his teaching:

> Gerdt taught beauty of line, expressiveness of movement, softness of *port de bras* (his pupils were famous for their arms), and, above all, a *cantilena* flow of dancing interwoven with acting. His memory held a real treasury of famous dances from the old repertory, which he used for the benefit of his pupils. He taught both men and women, strictly distinguishing between male and female grace. His men-pupils were masculine, while the ballerinas trained by Gerdt for ever retained a feminine softness and poise, coupled with beauty and perfection of *épaulement*.[14]

Christian Petrovitch Johannsen, who emphasized "strength, equilibrium, stamina, and correct breathing," was another teacher with whom Karsavina would study.[15] An old man by the time Karsavina knew him, he was, she recalled, a one-eyed Swede who "spoke broken Russian intermingled with French." His oaths were plentiful and his temper was fiery. Accompanying the class with his fiddle, he would frequently use the bow to point out her mistakes, and he once threw the bow at her, pronouncing her an "Idiot!" She recounts, "On the point of bursting into sobs, I turned my back and left the room. Segei [Legat] followed me. 'Come, angel, come and ask his pardon; the old man loves you. Be sensible.' He led me up to Christian Petrovitch. I apologised. For the first time I saw him smile. 'I taught your father,' he said to me. He took my hand; it was wet with perspiration. 'Clammy,' declared he, 'your blood wants purifying. Drink Hamburg tea.'"[16]

Mathilde Kschessinska, who graduated from the school in 1890, was older than Karsavina and thus knew a different Johannsen, and she describes his classes with reverence. She had entered Johannsen's class at the age of fifteen and returned to his class often throughout the years to benefit from his lessons in lyrical flow and elegance. Clearly not intimidated by the master,

Kschessinska described him as an excellent teacher, "a poet, an artist and inspired creator." "Every movement he made had meaning," she said, "expressed a thought, reflected a state of soul, which he strove to pass on to us."[17]

While Karsavina's success at the Imperial Ballet School seemed assured, her father's role as a teacher was threatened. In 1896 Karsavina's father lost his position at the school, although she returned as usual in August to begin her third term as a student. That year, she noted, several changes had been wrought in the curriculum. One of them was stimulated by the appearances in St. Petersburg of the Italian ballerina Pierrina Legnani. "In those days," Karsavina writes, "the engagement of a foreign star for a part of the season was customary."[18] Legnani distinguished herself as a dancer of great strength and virtuosity, introducing her *tours de force,* the "acrobatic" thirty-two fouettés. Although it resembled a circus trick, writes Karsavina, the stunt won over all critics by introducing an element of suspense: "Legnani walked to the middle of the stage and took an undisguised preparation. The conductor, his baton raised, waited. Then a whole string of vertiginous pirouettes, marvelous in their precision and brilliant as diamond facets, worked the whole audience into ecstasies. Academically, such an exhibition of sheer acrobatics was inconsistent with purity of style; but the feat, as she performed it, had something elemental and heroic in its breathless daring. It overwhelmed criticism."[19]

It may have been as a result of Legnani's great success, Karsavina said, that the school officials decided to offer a class in Italian technique taught by Maestro Enrico Cecchetti. Even Kschessinska, by this time a noted ballerina, went to Cecchetti to prepare herself "to attain the virtuosity which the Italian dancers were then demonstrating on the Russian stage." Italian technique, Kschessinska explains in her memoirs, "called for abrupt, precise, clear-cut movements, while Russian and French techniques are more lyrical, softer, more expressive, even in steps most marked with brio and virtuosity. It was only later that I was to return to our own technique, realising its grace and beauty."[20]

Though Karsavina would study diligently with Maestro Cecchetti once she went abroad with Diaghilev, in her last years of school both she and her father were happy to learn that she would not go to Cecchetti's class but to Gerdt's. It was taken as an honor that Gerdt had chosen Karsavina to be in his class when she was older. In the meantime, she worked "fanatically" in an intermediary class, earning the nickname "self-torturing fakir" from her classmates.[21]

Senior girls preparing to make their debuts underwent the scrutiny of their juniors, who were meanwhile anticipating their own graduations. As Cecchetti's training in physical strength and brilliant virtuosity was then in vogue, and as Legnani was clearly an audience favorite, all new *danseuses* were ranked according to their strength and bravura qualities. The fragile Anna Pavlova, who graduated in 1899, became the subject of heightened conversation among the students. Admittedly, Pavlova didn't have the admired body type, and she seemed so frail as to appear weak. "Romanticism was not the fashion any more," Karsavina explains, for the students uniformly preferred the compact, strong body type of Legnani and others who were built like her. "Pavlova at that time hardly realised that in her lithe shape and in her technical limitations lay the greatest strength of her charming personality," Karsavina adds.

> Meagreness being considered an enemy of good looks, the opinion prevailed that Anna Pavlova needed feeding up. She must have thought it, too, as she swallowed conscientiously cod-liver oil, the school doctor's panacea, and the aversion of us all. Like the rest of us, she strove to emulate the paragon of virtuosity, Legnani. Luckily for her, Guerdt fully divined the quality of her talent. It pained him to see executed by the delicate limbs of Pavlova what seemed consistent only with the hard set musculature of the Italian dancer. He advised her not to strive after the effects that seemed to endanger her frail structure.[22]

Though she does not dwell on the subject, Karsavina at times worked so hard and became so fatigued that she too became anemic and overly thin. Even during her period of ill-health, though, Karsavina fretted mainly that she would not be able to perform to her own high standards. Her mother was worried: "Mother, alarmed by my thinness, brought me some tonic wine. For a time I successfully hid it, now in my locker, now tucking the bottle under my shawl and secreting it in the school form. I had to give a dose of it to other girls, and the tonic, being sweet, diminished rapidly." The bottle was discovered by one of the matrons, who, "scandalised with what she concluded to be a vicious propensity," demanded an explanation from Karsavina's mother. A compromise was reached whereby the tonic could be stored in the infirmary and doled out as necessary. But, as a consequence for her secretive behavior, Karsavina was denied her regular Sunday leave and "there the incident ended." "I felt like a martyr then," she writes, but "in all justice, I must admit there was some foundation for the punishment."[23]

The strain of her family's increasing impoverishment must have taken a physical and emotional toll on Karsavina. Though she would be finished with her dance course in spring 1902, when she was seventeen, it was unprecedented for a girl to leave school before the age of eighteen. Nevertheless, Platon Karsavin was not earning a substantial living and Karsavina's mother pushed to have her daughter graduate early so she could contribute her dancer's salary to the family's meager income. But on Karsavina's return to school in the autumn of 1901, the matrons and school doctors pronounced that she appeared to be in worse health than before the summer break, and they voiced concerns about her ability to sustain a career as a dancer. "Nevertheless, I was getting stronger as time went on. Regular hours, plain wholesome food, airy rooms, periodical courses of tonic—the whole régime of the school helped me to overcome my anemia."[24]

In the end, those last two years of school were, she writes, "devotional and happy. . . . Full of a single purpose, every day revealed to me new heights to strive for." Her only concern, she says, was that the time remaining in school "might not be long enough to achieve all I wanted."[25] She knew that she had won the esteem of her teachers and, in spite of her doctors' concerns, in autumn 1901 she was given the coveted white dress, a mark of the highest distinction. In hindsight she realized that "the last years at school were a foretaste of the future career." Much of the energy and interest of the older dancers was centered on the emerging senior students, whose reputations were shaped even before they made their official debuts. "We stood in the anteroom of the stage, waiting to step in and conquer," writes Karsavina. "No thought of difficulties on the way to success ever crossed our minds."[26]

Finally at Lent, her mother was given the news that, as an exception, Karsavina was to be granted an early graduation. In spite of Karsavina's eagerness to finish school, the prospect of graduation terrified her: "I realised that my present means were inadequate to attain the high ideal I had set myself; I had thought to leave the school and appear on the stage equipped with full mastery; only much later did I understand that the stage is a school in itself, a cruel one perhaps, and at times unsparing, but the only school to temper the mettle of the artist's soul."[27]

Outside the walls of the Imperial Ballet School, the Russian empire was undergoing social upheaval to which the dancers would respond in due course. But at Karsavina's graduation, the ballet remained mostly insulated from the peasants' impoverished living conditions, the workers' strikes and student marches, and the rampant political assassinations. Linked to an outdated monarchical system, the world of the ballet seemed, in the words of Tim Scholl, an "aristocratic bauble."[28] Karsavina's world of the theater and its backstage life functioned within a city that itself appeared to be shut off from the "real" Russia experienced by many desperately impoverished Russians.

St. Petersburg was a spectacular construction with aristocratic origins;

created by tsars who looked to the West, the city had always been distinct from the "Russian-ness" of Moscow. Between 1796 and 1885, Alexander I and Nicholas I, grandsons of Catherine the Great, rebuilt St. Petersburg to suit the magnificence of what Bruce Lincoln has called a "colossal Eurasian empire" that "ruled more than a sixth of the land surface on the globe." Lincoln recounts, "Towering buildings modeled on the structures of ancient Rome replaced the more elegant, less pretentious ones from Catherine's time. Built during the first half of the nineteenth century, the Senate, the Synod, the Admiralty, the Ministry of War, the Headquarters of the General Staff, the Foreign Ministry, the Cathedrals of Our Lady of Kazan and St. Isaac, the Imperial Theaters—even the school of the Imperial Ballet—all called to mind the days when Rome had ruled the ancient world."[29]

The artist Alexandre Benois, one of the early collaborators in the initial ventures of the Diaghilev Ballets Russes, wrote of his city that "the greatest artists, writers, painters, musicians, lived in Peterburg and found inspiration there." He admitted that one who considered himself a "real" Russian might view the city as a "usurper"; however, Petersburg's original "mission" was to serve as a bridge to the West and, as such, the city was truly Russian in spirit and nature. "As the window on to Europe," he wrote, "it lit up the abode of the whole Russian people, though of course many varied foreign elements flocked to it owing to the very nature of its mission."[30]

Inside this city of grandeur and autocratic will, the Maryinsky Theatre invited spectators into a world of elegance, grace, and diversion. Benois describes the theater as a vast, airy auditorium designed for maximum visibility from every seat in the house. The decorations were "perfection": "True, the decorations, in the rococo style of Louis-Philippe, are not in fashion now, but nevertheless the style is extremely graceful and unobtrusive; the combination of blue hangings in the boxes, and the stalls and barriers upholstered in gold on a white background, create a harmony of remarkable gaiety and at the same time cosiness."[31]

Monarchical support for the ballet operated both on an official level and, in the case of Nicholas II, on a private level; prior to his coronation and his marriage to Princess Alix of Hesse-Darmstadt, Nicholas dedicated his love to the ballerina Mathilde Kschessinska. Inextricably woven into the tsar's daily life, the ballet and opera were also institutions of the imperial state. Garafola writes:

> Autocracy in Russia was not only sovereign, it was everywhere. Like an octopus, it spread its tentacles into preserves long since appropriated in Western

Europe by the private sector or given over to professionals. In the realm of cultural activity, particularly, state and tsar were synonymous. Institutions like the Imperial Academy of Arts and the Imperial theaters existed as departments under the jurisdiction of the Imperial court. They were funded by the Imperial Chancellery, which is to say, out of the tsar's own purse, and headed by relatives of the emperor or aristocrats personally appointed and responsible to him. To all intents and purposes, Imperial training academies and Imperial performance halls existed as fiefdoms of the Tsar of All the Russias.[32]

Nicholas Romanov dearly loved the opera, theater, and ballet. As a carefree youth, says Bruce Lincoln, "Nicholas saw Tchaikovsky's new *Sleeping Beauty* ballet three times in the month after its premiere. He dined, drank, sang, and danced night after night, often the whole night through, as he took in all the pleasures that the vibrant culture of Russia's great capital had to offer." As a young man, Nicholas was won over by Kschessinska, a "small and vivacious" beauty who was not yet eighteen, and whose career would flourish as their love did.[33] In the hierarchy that was the Imperial Ballet, Kschessinska was the Maryinsky's prima ballerina; she won the hearts of the tsar and of his cousins, Grand Duke Sergei Mikhailovich and Grand Duke Andrei Vladimirovich (whom she eventually married). As a consequence of her aristocratic associations, Kschessinska was, as Sally Banes puts it, inclined to "manipulate behind the scenes."[34] Kschessinska's rapid rise to power and fame was unprecedented, for the usual course of a dancer's ascent through the ranks was steady and sometimes slow.

Like Kschessinska, Karsavina was promoted rapidly instead of climbing slowly through the ranks, and her experience after graduation was compressed. As her father had predicted, Karsavina was soon drawn into the rivalry and political entanglements of the theater. Nevertheless, writes Karsavina, "The tedious grind through which many a dancer went before reaching any prominence had been spared me. From the very beginning I was placed amongst the chosen. My career began under good auspices. The policy of the new director [Vladimir Teliakovsky, appointed in 1902] was favourable to the young; every opportunity, every encouragement were given to those who showed any promise." However, older dancers warned that she should not be deceived by the encouragement. Nadejda Alexeievna, a friendly older dancer, warned her that "the theatre is a hotbed of intrigues."[35] Alexeievna, said Karsavina, "never aspired to any fame" herself and appeared to be well satisfied with her involvement in the ample social life of the theater. She was "indisputably elegant" but never hoped to reach further than the front line of the *corps de ballet*. Taking the younger woman under her wing, Alexeievna attempted to help Karsavina meet her "public," urging her to attend supper parties with balletomanes and critics. Alexeievna also strove to guard Karsavina from the jealousies of other ballerinas. When a renowned ballerina gave Karsavina a costume as a gift, Alexeievna responded skeptically: "Why do you think she made you a present of this costume?" Though Karsavina thought the costume particularly beautiful, Alexeievna cautioned her against wearing it, as she continued to harp, "Fancy you in dark mauve! . . . A pall for a coffin, not a costume for a child."[36]

Later, in writing her memoirs, Kschessinska attempted to clear up what she said was a misinterpretation, for she had been the famous ballerina in question. "In the spring of 1902 the delightful Tamara Karsavina graduated from the Ballet School, a beautiful girl, gifted, simple and full of infinite kindness," she wrote. Grand Duke Wladimir Alexandrovitch asked Kschessinska to take Karsavina under her wing and look after the young dancer's progress. "But Karsavina proved so gifted and so finished an artist that she had no need of my protection," Kschessinska said. "In the autumn of the same year, when she was to appear in a very difficult *pas-de-deux*, I gave her one of my own costumes, so that she might appear under the best conditions. . . . Pale blue and deep lilac were then the fashionable colours, two shades which were present in the costume I gave Karsavina."[37]

Duly warned about the potential jealousies of other dancers, Karsavina steadily pursued her work, still living at home, contributing to her family's meager income, and avoiding the "wickedness" of Alexeievna's supper parties. Yet, in spite of her evident achievements Karsavina still occasionally suffered from strain and overwork. Lacking sufficient self-confidence, she became "plagued by fears." Before the end of her first year on stage, however, the all-powerful ballet master Marius Petipa registered his approval by rewarding her with her first leading part, in a one-act ballet called *The Awakening of Flora*. The role was a pure dance role demanding a high level of virtuosity. "A year of Johannsen's rebukes had not been spent in vain," she claimed. "I could now master considerable difficulties."[38]

All went well until the actual rehearsals began. She recounted, "I must have overworked myself by that time, my toes were blistered, and my strength began failing me. The approach of the performance brought a sickening fear." Both well-wishers and rivals acted on her nerves. She recalled that "my friends on the stage wanted to impress me with the importance of success; some, less well-disposed, said it was much too early for me to have a responsible part. Both encouragement and discouragement were equally pernicious to my mental balance. Once the idea of possible failure had been put into my head, it began working ravages with my self-control. It hypnotised me. On the eve of my performance, some trivial discussion arose at home. I was highly strung; Mother lost her temper with me. I cried the best part of the night, and woke up in the morning with aching head and swollen eyes."[39] She felt queasy through the entire evening, and her memories of the performance were blurry. "At the end applause roared, and bouquets filled the stage. It didn't cheer me up; I had sentenced myself as a failure."[40]

In her third year, Karsavina became ill and was finally diagnosed with acute malaria. No doubt aware of the family's straitened circumstances, Kshessinska asked if she could help. But Karsavina noted, "I was grateful that Mother did not want to profit by her kind offer. A subsidy as well as a loan had been granted to me by the Chancery; that made it possible for Mother to take me abroad. Two months in Roncegno rid me of the fever." Having lost her hard-won technical strength, Karsavina was loath to return to Petersburg for the start of the fall season. She decided instead to take time to study with Signora Beretta, a popular teacher at La Scala in Milan. Both Vera Trefilova and Pavlova had demonstrated enormous progress after their studies with Beretta, and Karsavina wished to improve her strength and technique.

> The methods of Beretta were those of the Italian school, which does not care for individual grace of movements, but is implacable as to correctness of attitudes and *port de bras*. Exercises were set in the systematic pursuit of virtuosity; the class was forcible, not a second of rest allowed during the whole bar practice. The result of it for me was a considerable degree of endurance and amplitude of breath. It was hard at the beginning. I had been used to milder practice, and during my first lesson I fainted at the bar.[41]

Karsavina's industriousness and artistry were rewarded with "the summit of a dancer's ambition—the leading part in a five-act ballet." But with this honor, the demands on her only increased. She said, "Now, no more a precocious and petted child of the public, I had reached the stage where much was asked of me—the justification of the faith formerly given to me on credit. Exacting demands now replaced indulgence. I had to readjust my position, and found it difficult." She admitted, "Above all, I was not equipped with the practical sense. I was as unfit for scheming as for defending myself from the inevitable rebukes of jealousy." Though ambitious to excel in her career, Karsavina lacked a backup troupe of influential admirers. Nevertheless, she had won the very important favor and protection of the director, Teliakovsky.[42]

After several years of studying with Nicolai Legat, Karsavina made the difficult decision, in 1909, to leave his class and to seek out a female teacher, Yevgenia Sokolova, who had established her private studio in St. Petersburg.[43] It was a serious decision as she did not want Legat to question her loyalty—which was profound—but she acknowledged that she felt the need to study with a woman. The move to the new teacher proved to be timely, though, for soon after joining Sokolova's class, Karsavina was granted leading roles in *Swan Lake* and *Corsair*. "This latter part was considered an incontestable success of mine," she wrote. "I owed it greatly to Madame Sokolova."[44]

Sokolova was an old-fashioned teacher, Karsavina believed, in that she paid detailed attention to courtesies like curtain calls.[45] She also advocated celibacy for ballerinas, counseling them to commit their energies to class and the stage, and to exclude most extraneous elements of personal life. Her dedication to Karsavina's training was immense. She taught her the best way to tie the ribbons on her pointe shoes, instructed her how to spend the day before an evening performance, and fed her supper in the evenings after classes. Another of Sokolova's coups, according to Karsavina, was to win for her the friendship and esteem of the most important St. Petersburg dance critic, Valerian Svetlov. As Sokolova and Svetlov were personal friends, Sokolova taught the critic to appreciate the young dancer's "orthodoxy."[46] "It may have been a stroke of strategy on her part in order to make Svetloff take interest in my work, when Madame Sokolova borrowed of him a volume of Byron for me to get inspiration for the part of Medora," Karsavina wrote. "The poem gave me no direct bearing on the plot, which was greatly modified for ballet purposes; but it helped me by bringing a concrete vision of Medora to my imagination."[47]

Though she continued occasionally to be demoralized by her lack of self-confidence, she recognized that Svetlov's criticism was astute and well placed. The two became friends, and, through the years, she came to rely on his intelligent insights. Her debut as Medora in *Le corsaire*, she said, "stands out as a milestone on my way. Blind groping was left behind; I could now see my way clear down the long path to my ideal."[48]

Although Marius Petipa (c. 1818–1910) was the "all-powerful leader of the Petersburg ballet" and the dominant force in Russian ballet of the second half of the nineteenth century, he was technically in the employ of the tsar.[49] Upon his arrival at the Maryinsky Theatre, he served first as a dancer; he then became assistant ballet master and teacher, and then, with the retirement of Arthur Saint-Léon, ballet master of the Imperial Ballet. Born and trained in France, Petipa never learned to speak more than a few words of Russian—despite his fifty-six years of devotion to the Russian stage—for not only was St. Petersburg a highly cosmopolitan city, but the Russian ballet was founded on the French tradition of the *danse d'école*. Even if the generation coming of age with Karsavina challenged the conventions associated with the classical ballet, there was no doubt that ballet's French lineage was developed and brought to new heights in Imperial Russia.

Natalia Roslavleva has described the so-called Age of Petipa as "the product of an historical evolution and of circumstances and the taste of the times."[50] Petipa's ballets of the 1860s and 1870s "represent a choreographic response to nineteenth-century grand opera," Tim Scholl writes.[51] They were full-scale spectacles that unfolded over several hours, employing numerous dancers and hordes of walk-ons who carried elaborate stage properties. If these spectacles became, as is often charged, "formulaic" and "banal," it is useful to remember that during his long tenure over the Russian ballet, Petipa staged approximately seventy-five ballets for the imperial theaters and created dances for about thirty-six operas.[52]

Roslavleva writes that in Petipa's best works, he brought choreography to the "apex of achievement," executed by "a pleiad of brilliant artists." She describes Petipa as a "true disciple of Perrot," and says that, like his teacher, Petipa "preferred to deal with three-dimensional characters, being interested in portraying the emotional side of their psychology. The fact that as choreographer he by far surpassed his great teacher in the art of creating endless dance patterns, original *enchainements*, and *ballabili* was only to his credit. Petipa represented a new step in the development of the very art of making emotional content expressed both in dance and in music."[53]

In his finest works, such as *Sleeping Beauty*, *Raymonda*, or *La bayadère*, Petipa's choreographic vocabulary portrayed character and expressed emotion. It is also the case, however, as Scholl points out, that Petipa's works additionally emphasized ballet's visual component, a heightened visibility of the body made possible by centuries of developments in the classical *danse d'école*. "The ballet's emphasis of the human body's maximal legibility evolved as the Renaissance perspective stage was developed," Scholl writes. "The basic positions of ballet—feet and arms rotated outward from the body with limbs extended—make the dancers' movements maximally visible to the audience. The erect body, the leaps and jumps into the air, and the poses and movements executed high on the toes represent the ballet's conquest of vertical space on the new stage."[54]

Rather than the narrative elements stressed in the Romantic ballets, it was the emphasis on spectacle as well as the grace and elegance of the *danse d'école* tradition, the highlighting of bodily legibility and spatial patterning of the *corps de ballet*, and the contrapuntal weaving of ensembles and soloists that marked Petipa's choreographic inventiveness. But, by the time Karsavina graduated, the master's works had begun to seem dated. "Although Petipa stood high in the esteem of Imperial dancers," Garafola writes, "for the generation that came of age in the early years of the twentieth century, his artistic accomplishment belonged to the past."[55] Karsavina recalled that each ballet's subject was "treated like a peg on which to hang numerous ballabiles. Though his choreographic mastery never deserted Petipa, he had lost sight of the . . . inner motivation of the dance."[56] It was precisely this inner motivation that the younger choreographer Michel Fokine wanted to recover in his work.

Garafola describes Fokine's "call for authenticity" within the forms of the *danse d'école* as "both an integral part of his aesthetic and the focus of his many dissatisfactions with the Imperial Theaters. From the start his ideal was that of a naturalist."[57] Further, Fokine's momentum toward naturalism was "a galvanizing imaginative force that hurtled the artist into the real world[;] . . . taught him the empirical method of the scientist; and impressed upon him that art was a vehicle of social change." As a young man, Fokine was obsessed by painting, travel, and music. He ventured outside the narrow confines of the Imperial Ballet to seek opportunities to perform on the mandolin and balalaika with other musicians who cared about reviving Russian folk music.[58] Afire with the political energies of the day, Fokine perceived himself, and conducted himself, as a fomenter of long-overdue reforms.

In the early decades of the twentieth century, both outside and, in a muted fashion, inside the walls of the Imperial Theatre, the need for reform was strongly felt. In 1905, across Russia, there were spontaneous eruptions of dramatic revolutionary fervor, "involving millions of workers that paralyzed the entire Empire."[59] "In St. Petersburg," Bruce Lincoln writes, "virtually everyone stopped work. Factory workers, servants, postal workers, telegraph operators, janitors, and hackney drivers all walked off their jobs, as did bank clerks, shop clerks, and clerks in government offices. Doctors, lawyers, schoolteachers, university professors, even the entire corps de ballet of the great Imperial Mariinski Theatre—all joined the strike. There were no newspapers, no streetlights, no tramcars. Food and fuel soon began to grow scarce."[60]

As Garafola notes, "in the overall panorama of the Revolution, the dancers' strike is certainly a minor footnote." Still, "the event had a major impact on the genesis and aesthetics of the early Ballets Russes." The dancers' strike organized and consolidated those agents of change whose ideas would create an upheaval in the regime of the Imperial Ballet. With Fokine leading and three future Ballets Russes artists (Karsavina, Pavlova, and Nijinsky, the latter heading the student group) supporting him, the 1905 strike "transformed the company's dissidents into the makers of a choreographic secession."[61]

Though history has recorded Karsavina as a supporter of the movement for reform within the theater, she was no doubt principally aligned with Fokine through her personal loyalties to him and her confidence in him as an artist. In her memoirs she registered a decided ambivalence toward the political activities:

> The autumn of 1905, the autumn of the attempted revolution, I remember even now as a nightmare. A cruel October wind from the sea, chill, sleet, sinister hush in the town. For several days trams had not been running, the strike gaining rapidly. My heart was heavy as one night I was going home from a political meeting which we artists had held that day. I chose a roundabout way, avoiding pickets. My thin shoes let in water. My feet were numb, my mind bewildered. That artists, so conservative at heart, usually so loyal to the Court, of which we were a modest part, should have succumbed to the epidemic of meetings and resolutions seemed to me like treason. Meetings were being held everywhere; autonomy, freedom of speech, freedom of conscience, freedom of the printed word—even children at school were passing these resolutions. Whether in full conscience of the cause (I have reason to think it was not so) or following a few leaders, our troupe also put forward claims and chose twelve delegates to negotiate them. Fokine, Pavlova and myself were amongst them. Our President was a man from the ranks of the *corps de ballet*, a student at the University, a man of high integrity and limited vision.[62]

Explaining the artists' demands to her family was difficult because she was not sure that her convictions matched those of the others. In fact, the revolutionary meeting ran counter to her love for the theater and her loyalty to her upbringing: "And now, like repeating a lesson, I told them at home that we were going to ask for autonomy, choose our own Committee to decide artistic questions and questions of salary; do away with the methods of bureaucratic organization. My words sounded hollow to my own ears. 'So you are in arms against the Emperor who gave you an education, position, means of livelihood. Don't you go raising any standards. You will bring your art to a high level if you become a great artist,' summed up Mother."[63]

In the end, Karsavina would stand by Fokine, although she was sick at heart over the whole affair. Her sadness increased when she learned of the suicide, on October 16, of Sergei Legat, a beloved friend and fellow dancer in the reform movement. According to Garafola, a commission of enquiry was set up after the strikes to investigate the uprisings at the Imperial Theatres, and various activists were dismissed or "warned." Joseph Kchessinsky, the brother of Mathilde Kchessinska, was dismissed for his role in the strike, "although thanks to his sister's influence within the Imperial Court, he did not lose his pension." Pavlova was told to "desist from further trouble or suffer the consequences." Other artists were denied good roles or promotions. "Mild, to be sure, by tsarist standards," Garafola says, "these repressive actions nevertheless deepened the rift between dissidents and management loyalists."[64]

The political and creative activities of the younger, reform-minded generation—including Fokine, Karsavina, Pavlova, Lydia Kyasht, and Vera Fokina—were inextricably connected, according to Garafola, who calls the Maryinsky a "microcosm of [the tsarist] society at large." The dancers' impulse toward change touched on all aspects of their dance lives: "It colored attitudes toward the 'old classical technique' epitomized by Kchessinska and Nicholas Sergeyev, the Imperial Ballet's chief regisseur, as well as the careerism such traditionalists represented." It also politicized Fokine's creative efforts and "sharpened criticism of the 'parasites of art,' as Fokine termed the officeholders who controlled the fortunes of the Imperial Theaters, impelling him and like-minded colleagues to seek work outside the bureaucratic world."[65]

Although Karsavina may have been heartsick at appearing disloyal to the tsarist system that had given her her training, she did strongly support Fokine in his artistic beliefs. The Michel Fokine she knew was forceful, at times intolerant, antagonistic, impetuous, and enthusiastic. But, "my belief in him was deeply rooted before he actually began producing," she wrote. "Through casual remarks of his, through tirades steeped with a feeling of a crusade to be led against the smug and the Philistine, there loomed new shores, there called glorious exploits."[66]

Fokine's call for reforms in ballet cohered around his belief that a ballet could represent an artistic wholeness. As a young man Fokine railed against the customary ways of the stage, which he believed stultified the art form and prevented choreographers from exploring expressive potentialities of the ballet. While the classical ballet training was ideal, he wrote, such training should make the body a versatile, expressive instrument and not simply cater to a public that craved virtuosity. He held that

> a straight back is ideal for a foundation. . . . But to build the entire form of the dance around a straight back is an error. Similarly with turned-out legs: if one did not sufficiently prepare oneself with the exercises of turning out, then the toe during dancing would have a tendency to turn in, and this is very ugly. But is it proper to substitute one ugliness for another? The exercise of turning out is, in fact, a very useful procedure. The legs are thus prepared to assume the most versatile positions and become flexible and obedient parts of the dancer's instrument—his body. . . . But the form of the dance should not be built on turned-out legs. Esthetically such a position is unacceptable.[67]

Fokine's process as a choreographer was imbued with a strong sense of history, and he defied tradition in urging that the dance vocabulary, costume, and action of a ballet should conform to the time period and locale portrayed. For Fokine, says Garafola, "empirical observation and research must accompany the act of creation," and a work's "expressiveness stemmed directly from the fidelity of [its] representation to nature."[68] In his memoirs, Fokine listed his grievances with what he considered Petipa's formulaic approach: "The dancer did not change his dance and manners in order to create the image of a certain period. On the contrary, all periods, all styles, all characters were subordinated to the dance, which was invariably in the same form. Everything was sacrificed for one form, one style, so that the artists might display the dance, the technique, in the manner in which it had been prepared—once and for all." There was no "transformation," he said, "no creation of an image. Instead self-exhibition." Applause interrupted the flow of the dancing and thus, in the Petipa ballet, there was no effort at creating a sense of "unity of action."[69]

In spite of her enormous regard for Fokine, Karsavina found that in their working relationship she sometimes had difficulty shedding "the beliefs in which [she] had been brought up."[70] For his part, Fokine did not have much to say about her role in bringing his ballets to life. He acknowledged that she was the ideal interpreter of the ballerina doll in *Petrouchka* and that her performance of the waltz from *Les sylphides* demonstrated "that rare romanticism" he was never able to evoke from later performers.[71] Nevertheless, though he was mostly silent about her participation, she was undoubtedly one of the chief interpreters of his ballets, taking leading roles in the ballets he created outside the auspices of the Maryinsky Theatre, prior to his work with Diaghilev, and in most of the new works created during his tenure as choreographer for the Ballets Russes.

Karsavina later spoke at length about her admiration for Fokine and her confidence in his work. She told John Drummond that Fokine was the first to understand that "ballet as it stood then couldn't develop any more. And he guessed from the great possibilities that were in the academic technique that it could develop, evolve. He created different styles of ballet, because he believed that every subject must have its own treatment and its own style, but they were all on the basis of the academic technique, only he went further without breaking with it."[72] Fokine's irascibility made him difficult to work with, she admitted, but the two worked so closely for so many years that finally she was able to interpret what he wanted before he had actualized the movement himself:

He had terrific tempers. Sometimes he would even throw chairs about. But withal very lovable. We were devoted to him, because he took the artists with him. He gave them insight into the part. Just to watch him dance in front of us. He was a magnificent dancer himself, and he would, as he danced in front, give a sort of running commentary on it. When he was angry, he would say, "It's putrid, tatty," but he could also admire the artists as he worked with them. He could stand back and say, "That's wonderful." And from my knowledge of him, working with him (as you know, I had all the leading parts in his ballets), I got to know him, and in a way anticipate what he wanted, and sometimes I would take a pose and he would say, "That's it, that's what I wanted."[73]

There were personal affiliations, too, between the handsome, passionate choreographer and the beautiful, intelligent dancer. "Everyone knew," Lydia Lopoukhova told Richard Buckle, that early in their careers "the budding choreographer and the not-yet ballerina had loved each other."[74] Lopoukhova who was, according to Buckle, "always fascinated by other people's private lives," once asked Karsavina why she had not married Fokine. The simple response was, "My mother did not think it would be a good idea." Karsavina's mother had married a dancer and wanted to spare her daughter that same economic uncertainty.[75] Instead, Fokine married another dancer who became known by her married name, Vera Fokina. And Karsavina took as her first husband Vassily Moukhin, a balletomane and violinist who worked in the Ministry of Finance.[76]

In the introduction to his book *Natasha's Dance,* Orlando Figes writes that "there is a Russian temperament, a set of native customs and beliefs, something visceral, emotional, instinctive, passed on down the generations, which has helped to shape the personality and bind together the community." It was this "Russian temperament" and "personality" that contributed to the "myth of exotic Russia," first carried to the West by the Ballets Russes.[77] Karsavina described much the same phenomenon in her memoirs: "The summer of 1909 saw the invasion of Russian art into Europe, Western Europe I should have said to be correct. Any Russian, speaking spontaneously, would have said 'Europe' to designate the countries to the west of our frontier, but instinctively we set ourselves apart." Isolated and mysterious as a nation, Russia had an art and culture that seemed unfathomable to most Western Europeans. "The whole of our vast country to the average occidental mind still remained a land of barbarians. Russia, crude and refined, primitive and sophisticated, the country of great learning and appalling ignorance."[78]

Since Russian art was rarely seen outside the country's borders, Karsavina and others in her circle were intrigued by the news that Serge Diaghilev had begun to introduce Russian art to the West. By 1908 the assertive and persuasive Diaghilev had taken an exhibition of eighteenth-century Russian portraiture to Paris, organized the art journal *Mir iskusstva* (The World of Art), and presented the "first *Boris Godunov* seen outside Russia."[79] Karsavina initially encountered the striking-looking impresario when she was fifteen and was taking a break in the rehearsal of *The Nutcracker.* In the coming years, she writes, "every new manifestation of his remarkable personality" would envelop her in "the aura of [his] genius." She was drawn to each of Diaghilev's new initiatives and attended all of the *Mir isskustva* exhibitions. She was intrigued by the fabled inner circle of his collaborators, and she longed to "penetrate into that holy of holies, where now they all worked together. Fokine would drop a word now and then relative to these artistic sittings at Diaghileff's flat. I stood wistfully outside the circle."[80] Diaghilev first visited her apartment to invite her to dance in his group of dancers on a tour to Paris, and it was a momentous and life-changing occasion. She would not comprehend its full importance until years later, though at the time she was most worried what Diaghilev, "the aesthete," might think of her.[81]

The role of Diaghilev's troupe in reintroducing ballet to the West was enormous. As Garafola puts it, Diaghilev managed to create "a company unique in the annals of European dance history, a massive entrepreneurial undertaking carried out in the name of beauty, imagination, and taste."[82] Further, there were significant connections between Diaghilev's Ballets Russes and the legacy of the Maryinsky Ballet, for the dancers in Diaghilev's troupe exhibited the professionalism, discipline, and reverence for the art form that had been imbued in them by their schooling:

> However much they may have inveighed against Maryinsky artistic policies
> ... the [Imperial Theatre] left a permanent mark on Diaghilev and his col-
> leagues. The high standard of professionalism that from the first distinguished
> Ballets Russes productions was an enduring Maryinsky legacy. Another was
> the conviction that ballet belonged in the opera house, that it was an art of
> high lyric theater. This meant that so long as Diaghilev had the means (and
> even when he did not), the scale of production was lavish, the setting the
> most prestigious he could muster; always he aspired to elevate the Ballets
> Russes to the status of a major operatic attraction. At the Maryinsky, ballet
> was inseparable from the substance and form of hereditary aristocracy. In the
> West, Diaghilev summoned a different, but no less powerful elite to the side
> of ballet—an aristocracy of money and taste.[83]

For Karsavina, those first months of her association with the Diaghilev Ballets Russes in Paris were unforgettable. "The fortnight preceding our performances [were] arduous, feverish, hysterical," she recalled. The Châtelat Theatre was "well-nigh shaken to its foundations by the tornado of what was to be the first Russian season in Paris. The stage hands, gruff as they only can be in Paris, the administration pedantic and stagnant, regarded us all as lunatics."[84] Sergei Grigoriev, who served as Diaghilev's *régisseur* (rehearsal director) from 1909 until the company's dispersal at Diaghilev's death in 1929, evoked the excitement of the evening, describing the premiere performance on May 19, 1909, as "a great day in the history of the Russian Ballet of Sergey Pavlovich Diaghilev." "All of us," wrote Grigoriev, "Diaghilev included, were at the theatre from early morning, and all in a feverish state. . . . The house was packed. There was not one empty seat. A few minutes before the curtain went up, Diaghilev appeared on the stage to address the dancers, who were all assembled. All Paris, he said, was there to see them and he wished them luck. Then, after asking me whether everything was ready, and being assured it was, he ordered the house lights to be dimmed; and the performance began."[85] The next day, the *régisseur* recalled, "the Russian Ballet was the talk of Paris."[86] To her surprise, Karsavina said, the newspapers informed her she had been dubbed "La Karsavina."[87]

After Diaghilev's Paris season Karsavina was offered a contract to dance at the London Coliseum. She was inclined to accept the opportunity to appear in London, she said, because the city attracted her fancy, and "I did so love Dickens at school." Impresario Marinelli arranged her appearances and set her up in a Leicester Square hotel. But once there, the reality of the obligation set in; she knew no one in London and spoke no English, and the contract she had signed demanded two performances a day, a rigorous schedule that positively terrified her.[88] She found that unlike the regimen at the Maryinsky, which required two performances a week, with plenty of time for rest and thorough rehearsal, in London she would appear as a "number" on a variety bill of diverse attractions.

All in all, Karsavina's first trip to London was difficult. In spite of the pioneering efforts of the Danish ballerina Adeline Genée to "fight the strong remains of Victorian prejudice" with her performances at the Empire Theatre, ballet was an unknown and undervalued art form in England.[89] Furthermore, conditions were not adequate for ballet, and the stage at the Coliseum was terrible. Nor, Karsavina said, was it possible to ensure that she would get sufficient rest. She recalled that it was "an extremely hard floor and the unavoidable brass bruised my toes and made them bleed. My first week was hardly over, and I dreaded the remaining three. Worse than my blistered toes was to me the feeling of not belonging anywhere in my present surroundings. I bore a grudge against the stained windows of the restaurant in my hotel, the noisy barrel-organ in the side street; it played in the morning, it played in the afternoon when I came to rest between performances."[90] She suffered most, however, from the loneliness as she watched the various music hall "numbers" depart on a weekly basis, only to be replaced by other performers with new variety acts. On the other hand, she said, everyone wanted to be kind to her; her dresser taught her a few words of English and Sir Oswald Stoll offered to double her salary to prolong her contract. But she was still thoroughly miserable, until one day Marinelli came through with the gift of a little King Charles spaniel. She named the dog Loulou and he became her constant companion.

The personal relationship between Vaslav Nijinsky and Diaghilev is one of the more mythologized aspects of the early Ballets Russes history. As Diaghilev recognized and nurtured Nijinsky's talents, the landscape for the male dancer changed dramatically, so that, as in the eighteenth century, the male dancer once again dominated the ballet stage. However, while Vestris's virility was said to have drawn women admirers, in the early years of the twentieth century Nijinsky's feline exoticism drew a strongly homosexual audience. "Diaghilev's heroes," Garafola writes, "traced a spectrum of male roles that transcended conventions of gender while presenting the male body in a way that was frankly erotic."[91] In the pre–World War I years, the *danseuse* receded from prominence on the ballet stage, and leading roles were given over to men. Ballet after ballet celebrated the male physique, "dramatized its athletic prowess, and paraded its sexual availability."[92]

In Diaghilev's domain, the chief roles were frequently devised to show Nijinsky's vast talents, accompanied by Karsavina as his ideal partner. While in the first season only *Cléopâtre* (1909) evinced the "shift in the [gender] paradigm," there were to be many more occasions for Nijinsky to dominate as hero of the ballet.[93] In 1910 Fokine created *Schéhérazade*; in 1911 there followed *Le spectre de la rose*, *Petrouchka*, and *Narcisse*; and in 1912 he choreographed (among other works) *Le dieu bleu* and *Thamar*, while Nijinsky began his own choreographic venture with the 1912 *L'après-midi d'une faune*, in which he himself performed as lead dancer.

Though each of these ballets featured choice roles for Nijinsky, it was widely acknowledged that Karsavina invested her roles with profound conviction and beauty. *Petrouchka*, Arnold Haskell writes, "revealed Nijinsky in a new light—as an actor of intense power."[94] In the role of the empty-headed ballerina,

Karsavina confirmed her fame. Peter Lieven described Nijinsky's portrayal of the puppet as "one of the most vivid and unforgettable impressions I have ever experienced." But Karsavina was, Lieven said,

> quite on the level of her wonderful partner. Her physical appearance was a great aid in this. She was a beautiful woman, and, by the use of make-up, her charming face was changed into the soulless plaster mask of a doll. Her technique and lightness of movement were perfect. She was the complete image of an empty, stupid, beautiful woman—a soulless, thoughtless doll. Karsavina's strength never lay in her temperament, and her classical style of dancing suited this part to perfection. The clarity, the plastic beauty and airy lightness of her movements gave her dance great freshness and a charming unreality.[95]

The rapidly conceived *Le spectre de la rose* proved to be what Lieven calls "one of Fokine's finest improvisations." Haskell says that the ballet, which was suggested by Jean Louis Vaudoyer after a poem by Gautier, was devised as a contrast to the rest of the program, particularly as a contrast for Nijinsky after his dramatic role in *Petrouchka*. This miniature ballet is a *pas de deux* for Karsavina, as a young girl returning from a ball, and Nijinsky, as the spirit of her rose. Nijinsky's dramatic leap out the girl's bedroom window near the end of the ballet, Haskell writes, "has passed into history, and has often made the audience forget the true climax of the little drama—the awakening and the gradual disillusionment of the young dreamer." Haskell was touched by Karsavina's role in the ballet: "No one has ever rendered it so exquisitely as Karsavina. It remains hers for ever."[96] Meanwhile, Lieven thought she was "quite worthy of the genius of her partner." There was something appealingly feminine about Karsavina, he said: "The expression of the 'eternal feminine' was particularly congenial to the talent of this delightful ballerina. The image of girlhood created by her was graceful, innocent, and poetical. Her dream-dance had a quiet, virginal, romantic charm."[97] According to these critics, Karsavina was appealingly feminine and a complement to the charismatic Nijinsky. While these viewers did not deny her magnificent artistry, however, they clearly ranked her as second fiddle.

Initially, the female roles in both *Giselle* and *Firebird* were intended for Pavlova, but they were given to Karsavina after Pavlova left Diaghilev to pursue her own engagements around the world. According to Grigoriev, it was Walter Nouvel who reminded Diaghilev that the male solo in *Giselle* would give Nijinsky the opportunity to demonstrate his classical technique.[98] Despite the Parisian audience's cool response to the production, and Diaghilev's initial reluctance to stage what first seemed an outdated and uninteresting ballet, Karsavina entered her rehearsals with Nijinsky with great seriousness and reverence:

"So intent were Nijinsky and I on making masterpieces of our respective parts in *Giselle*, that our eagerness to impose on one another our individuality led to tempestuous scenes. *Giselle*, on our stage, was a holy ballet, not a step of it to be altered. I knew the part as taught me by Madame Sokolova, and loved every bit of it. I was sadly taken aback when I found that I danced, mimed, went off my head and died of broken heart without any response from Nijinsky. He stood pensive and bit his nails." Their difficulties in accommodating each other's interpretations led to tears and fury. From that moment on, Karsavina said, Diaghilev "acted as a buffer between us."[99]

Firebird was the "big" creation for 1910, and it too was originally conceived for Pavlova as the Firebird with Fokine as the Prince. However, in the long run, it was the role of the Firebird, says Haskell, that first gave Karsavina her world fame. "No one could have interpreted [the role] more perfectly than did Thamar Karsavina. For her it was the ideal part, a combination of drama and classicism in which her remarkable beauty could be seen to full advantage."[100] With her vast reserves of artistry and talent, Karsavina excelled in the roles she had learned in school and in those Fokine created for her. Nonetheless, even she was to be eclipsed by Nijinsky.

Patience was one of Karsavina's many strengths. Garafola explains that there was a steady stream of ballerinas who came and went from Diaghiev's company when it became clear that their scope and ambitions as classical dancers would not be fulfilled. Only Karsavina remained consistently loyal to Diaghilev, though "by 1913 she had become sufficiently restive to demand a work of her own." The ballet promised to her was *La tragédie de Salomé*, which "was sufficiently minor that it would not detract from the season's other premiers: Nijinsky's *Jeux* and his monumental *Le sacre du printemps*. Unsurprisingly, the fillip endured for no more than a season."[101]

In 1911 Vaslav Nijinsky was fired from the Maryinsky Theater, which left him free to remain with Diaghilev fulltime. From then on Diaghilev's insistent demands that Karsavina sign a long-term contract with him increased in volubility. She was reluctant to take more work with Diaghilev, however, because she was already carrying a heavy share of the repertory at the Maryinsky and treasured her increasingly rare rest periods. In 1910 Karsavina had been given the title of prima ballerina at the Maryinsky, and she was offered a renewable contract that provided her a larger salary than her relatively few years in the service of the tsar would otherwise command. Diaghilev knew that although the number of her performances was stipulated by contract, she was free to choose the times when she would perform at the Maryinsky and was liberally granted leaves of absence. The terms of her contract prompted him to increase his pressure on her when, in fact, she said, "my work in Petersburg was intensified, compressed into a shorter period."[102] As Diaghilev pestered her she grew increasingly unsettled by his demands: "Indeed, I saw dangerous signs in the rapidly increasing volume of Diaghileff's ambitions. As, enlarging his enterprise, he wanted more and even more of my time, we became constantly engaged in unequal struggles. Exhortations from him, ineffectual arguments from me—he would win at the end. Neither could I sever myself from his work, I loved it, nor would he spare me."[103]

Why did Karsavina remain loyal to Diaghilev when she clearly had many other options? According to the ballerina herself, it was because she had an implicit belief in him and his artistic project. She described Diaghilev as having "enlarged the scope of my artistic emotions; he educated and formed me, not by ostentatious methods, not by preaching or philosphising. A few casual words fetched a lucid conception, an image to be, out of the dark."[104] Until she left Diaghilev's troupe finally in 1920, Karsavina would juggle her obligations at the Maryinsky (which ended in 1918), her performances with Diaghilev, and her own European engagements. Garafola explains that for Karsavina, the choice finally to sever ties with Diaghilev was both an artistic and an economic decision. The ballerina "'broke' with Diaghilev in 1920 for artistic reasons. Among the newer ballets few roles offered scope for dramatic expression or demanded the strong classical technique of the ballerina who had reigned over the Maryinsky no less than the prewar Ballets Russes. Karsavina, moreover, did not need Diaghilev. As a star on whom offers poured from managements all over Europe, she enjoyed both the luxury of independence and a level of monetary reward Diaghilev could afford only at intervals."[105]

In an article she wrote decades later entitled "Why the 'Ballet Russe' Could Not Survive Diaghileff," Karsavina reminisced about her relationship with the charismatic impresario. She was aware of his foibles. His constant searching after new art forms and his seeming rejection of classical ballet had prompted her to leave the company in 1920. In retrospect, though, she continued to admire his passionate convictions. Diaghilev's intent was not simply to create fads, she said. Instead, he was motivated by "the passionate belief that art should never become crystallised into any form of classicism but must develop as a living organism, finding in the process of its growth new, fresh modes of expression to translate the new thoughts, the new discoveries of the human intellect." She defended his adherence to classicism, which many others questioned: "In fact, he respected tradition and valued its technical achievements: nothing short of perfect technique would satisfy him, whatever the style of a production." He also demonstrated an "unerring judgment of artistic values" and an amazing capacity to organize. She also noted that he often strained the "physical endurance of his artists" and "rarely failed to have his own way with all those around him."[106]

So it was that Karsavina continued to honor her obligations to Diaghilev's troupe as well as those at the Maryinsky. In her relentless schedule, Haskell says, she was "practically taking off her make-up on the train as she journeyed from Saint Petersburg to the West and lived her double life. It required enormous effort of mind and body, only possible in one extremely adaptable."[107]

Adaptability, versatility, and intelligence: these are the characteristics frequently mentioned in descriptions of Karsavina's approach to her work. To Lieven she was "more highly cultured than the average ballerina." She was distinctly not like Pavlova, "with whom one could not talk except in a half-coquettish ballet fashion," he said. Instead, "Karsavina was capable of sustaining a serious conversation."[108] Her second husband was also awestruck by her intelligence. Her mind, Bruce said, "was stored with a profound knowledge of the history and background of all branches of the art of the theatre; stored too with an encyclopaedic familiarity with Russian, French and, even, English literature; with a memory rivalling Macaulay's, so that she could read a long poem once, shut the book and recite it without fault or hesitation."[109] Bruce maintained there were two Tamaras. "The home one lived largely in the clouds, in a world where time meant nothing, where much of it was spent in the almost hourly search for objects which she had a genius for mislaying." The Tamara who inhabited the theater, though, had both feet on the ground. In the theater, "time had a meaning and a very precise one. Two hours to the minute before the curtain should go up, she would be in her dressing-room to get everything, including her mind, ready for the performance. . . . woe betide anybody then, in those two hours, who broke in upon her thoughts with chatter."[110]

The evidence of her life suggests that Karsavina knew how to get her feet on the ground outside the theater more than Bruce admitted. Prior to their marriage, for instance, she recognized that she loved him and set about securing a divorce from her first husband. "When [Bruce] came into her life it was obvious that she had fallen in love with him, and Moukhin put his own interests on one side and, refusing to stand in the way of her happiness, gave her a divorce," according to Peter Lieven.[111] Buckle reports that Karsavina's former in-laws thought she "treated Moukhin very badly by deserting him for Bruce." He added, "It was the only time I ever heard anyone say a word against her."[112]

She could take care of herself in the frightening aftermath of the Russian Revolution, too. In *Theatre Street* she described an instance when she stood up to soldiers who arrived to search her flat:

> On the first anniversary of the Revolution, manifestations were held in the town, processions moved about. One was safer indoors. The day before, I had had a dispute with our Commissar on behalf of the company. My husband said, "You'd better be careful." Hardly had he spoken when we heard a scuffle outside, sound of many feet running upstairs; my door resounded with heavy blows. On the landing stood a group of soldiers; my husband's warning seemed to have come true. My fear suddenly changing into irritation, I spoke angrily to them, and the soldiers, amazingly mild and even confused, explained that they were searching for the porter who might be hiding in my flat. He apparently had offended them by an ironical remark. On my assurance that I was not hiding him, the soldiers went off.[113]

On May 15, 1918, Karsavina performed *La bayadère* for the close of the Maryinsky season. It would be the last time she would dance in Russia. The British Embassy had closed in February and Bruce had left her behind with their son. He was not able to return to Russia until June to conduct her and two-year-old Nik out of the country. Then, everything seemed to go awry.

First there were difficulties obtaining the needed British passports, and once en route, they were warned of possible interference from Bolshevik commissars, who were suspicious of all English nationals. The family chose to continue their evacuation anyway and found a small boat that took them secretly to a remote village. There, sympathetic peasants donated horse-drawn carts to allow the evacuees to continue their escape, and Karsavina was forced to discard all but the necessary belongings. "We drove for a whole week through dense forests by innumerable lakes with deep and dark water. No towns, the villages far apart—the country cheerless, sinister," she wrote. Meanwhile her terrified child clutched at her dress and "cried and screamed day and night. He slept but occasionally; at times my knees grew numb under his weight, but the slightest movement of mine would set him screaming and clutching desperately at me."[114]

At last, their horse carts arrived in a more prosperous village, which had a soviet. Karsavina recognized there was trouble ahead when some drunken peasants approached them without removing their caps and accused Karsavina and Bruce of forging their passports. She knew then, she said, that her husband's mild-mannered approach would not work with these men: "I picked up Nikita and came out: the offensive alone could save the situation. My husband described my attitude as that of a tiger cat. Our passports certainly were dubious pieces of paper, but fortunately I remembered that there was another document in my husband's pocket, quite irrelevant now, a pass to Moscow dated some months ago. . . . With this in my hand, I bluffed, threatening to report them for disregarding the orders of their government, and called them a name or two."[115]

When they finally arrived in England, Bruce and family were sent by the Foreign Office to Tangier, a place for a "perfect rest cure." Bruce recalled, "The war years at our Embassy in Russia had been all so grilling, the year of Revolutions and of our escape such an unremitting nightmare that I begged the Foreign Office for a quiet post where we could all three regain our balance, for Nik too during our flight had been mad with subconscious terror."[116] Life in Tangier was serene, said Bruce, until the telegrams started arriving from Diaghilev, demanding that Karsavina return to the Ballets Russes to dance in the upcoming season in London. She could not resist his pleas. "In fact, these negotiations were a true reflection of the essential difference in their outlook upon life," wrote Bruce. "To Diaghileff, home life meant just nothing. He had no home and didn't want one. The ballet was his all in all, the ballet and the arts that served it. There was only one Diaghileff. There were two Tamaras—the Karsavina of the theatre, the Tamara of the home. In the constant struggle that went on round these two aspects of her life the impresarios pulled one way, Tamara pulled the other."[117]

At many points in her married life, though, Karsavina needed the additional income from her dancing to provide for her family as Bruce left the diplomatic service to try his hand, first, at painting. His venture as an artist was not successful, however, and he recognized that "I was not pulling my weight in our pair-oar, just 'sugaring' as rowing men say. Tamara's blade was doing all the work. That must stop. I would turn to commerce or finance."[118] He was no more happy, or financially secure, in recreating himself as a banker, so he then took an assignment in Bulgaria with the official title of Secretary General to the British Delegation of the Interallied Reparations Commission, for vastly more money than he had been making at the bank. Karsavina continued her whirlwind touring. In a letter from Hamburg in October 1921, she wrote to Bruce, "I have a matinée here at 11.30. To-night I go to Munich. Will be back in Hamburg Wednesday morning and will dance for Russian people, artists and so on, who could afford buying tickets. Thursday another matinée if they can find a theater. Sunday I go to Prague. There is an offer for Copenhagen and several for Sweden." Bruce knew the misery she was enduring. During those years, he said, she spent approximately six months "touring, mostly in Germany; once in America and Canada."

They were times for her of the acutest misery; of utter loneliness and yet of longing to be left alone; of poignant homesickness; of a tiredness, less even of body than of mind, which was hardly to be borne. The day would come, she knew, when she would rejoin Nik and me, resuming the picnics and the pottering life she loved. Meanwhile, there was a vista of weary months to be sighed and sometimes wept through—months of constant travel, and that as a rule by night; of rehearsals next morning; of never-ending worries over money and exchange; of all difficulties with agents and with tiresome dancing partners; of all the hundred and one things that make a touring dancer's life a purgatory.[119]

Finally, in 1926 the family left their post in Sofia, Bulgaria, and returned to London, where they bought a house in the Albert Road with a view of Regent's Park. There Karsavina taught in a little studio she had opened just off Baker Street, wrote her memoirs, and made guest appearances here and there. She continued to inspire and impress other dancers. For example, her influence on the young British choreographer Frederick Ashton was enormous:

I remember my alarm at being allowed to touch her, let alone partner her, knowing that she had danced with all the great of her generation. Her attitude towards me was one of complete patience and encouragement, nevertheless demanding my absolute dedication and understanding of the technicalities of the roles. They were days of inspiration and absorption on my part, and the knowledge I acquired of the real meaning of dancing was invaluable for my future work. I drenched myself in her presence—I learnt the meaning of gesture, "nuance," the drama of movement inherent in the dance—and, watching her performance, the immense importance of the *"épaulement,"* now almost a lost aspect in most dancers.[120]

KARSAVINA'S CONTINUED INFLUENCE

Mary Clarke explains that Karsavina assisted the Royal Academy of Dancing in London in devising its Teacher's Training Course and had served the organization as a vice president for a time.[121] Karsavina was well suited for her role in helping to develop the academy's pedagogy. In her book *Ballet Technique: A Series of Practical Essays,* Karsavina describes the slow and systematic training that she received at the Imperial Theatre School in St. Petersburg. The book is primarily intended for teachers, who, she says, must be attentive to the problems that occur in training and who must be creative in finding remedies for mistakes that creep into the student's practice. She cites her favorite teachers, Sokolova and Gerdt, and describes special exercises each would give for strengthening *adage* work (Sokolova) and increasing *ballon* (Gerdt), thus contributing to the transmission of the Russian ballet tradition to the West.

Karsavina's influence was invoked when I attended a conference that coincided with the American Ballet Theatre company's new production of Frederick Ashton's *La fille mal gardée*. Ashton's ballet, choreographed in 1960, was based on the Jean Dauberval 1786 original, first performed in Bordeaux. The conference I attended included a talk by the former Royal Ballet dancer Sir Alexander Grant, who had coached the American Ballet Theatre dancers in their new production. Grant reminded his audience that it was Karsavina who encouraged Ashton to choreograph his version of the ballet. Her role as Lise in that ballet had been one of her favorites back in St. Petersburg. While working with Ashton, Karsavina recalled the ballerina Virginia Zucchi's late nineteenth-century performances of the ballet and taught Ashton her beloved mime scene in the ballet's second act.

That night as I watched the tiny Russian-born ballerina Nina Ananiashvili in the ballet choreographed by Ashton, an Englishman, and staged for the American Ballet Theatre company, based in New York, my thoughts drifted across geography and through time. I watched Lise act out, through traditional gesture language, her centuries-old dream of a future with her beloved Colas, and I felt Karsavina's presence.

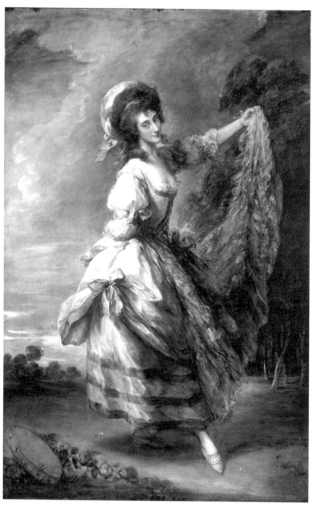

Thomas Gainsborough. Giovanna Baccelli
in *Les amans surpris,* (choreography by
Simonet), 1782. Tate Gallery, London /
Art Resource, N.Y.

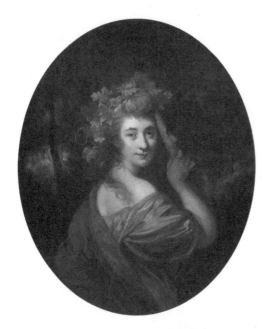

J. R. Smith. Mademoiselle Baccelli. Engraving of a portrait by Sir Joshua Reynolds, 1783. Jerome Robbins Dance Division; New York Public Library for the Performing Arts; Astor, Lenox, and Tilden Foundations.

Adèle Dumilâtre as Myrtha in *Giselle* (choreography by Coralli and Perrot), 1843. Jerome Robbins Dance Division; New York Public Library for the Performing Arts; Astor, Lenox and Tilden Foundations.

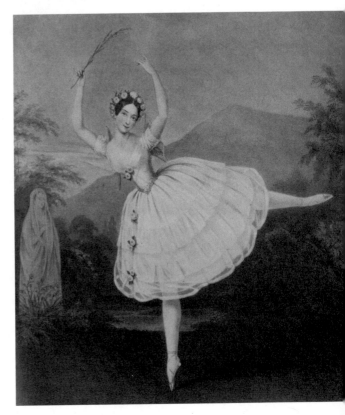

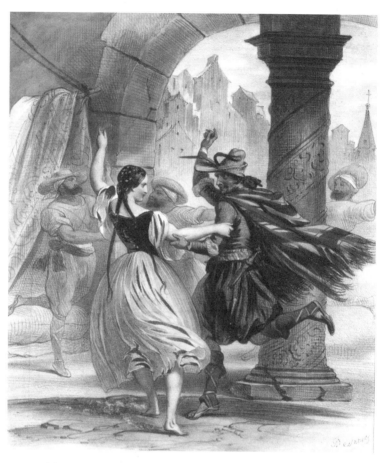

Adèle Dumilâtre in *La gypsy,* act 2
(choreography by Mazilier), 1845[?].
Jerome Robbins Dance Division; New
York Public Library for the Perform-
ing Arts; Astor, Lenox and Tilden
Foundations.

Adèle Dumilâtre in *La polka*
(choreographer unknown),
1844. Jerome Robbins Dance
Division; New York Public
Library for the Performing
Arts; Astor, Lenox and Tilden
Foundations.

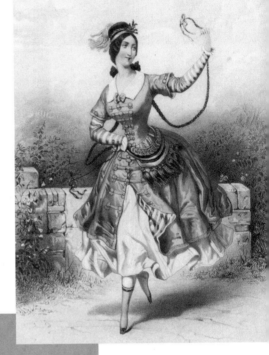

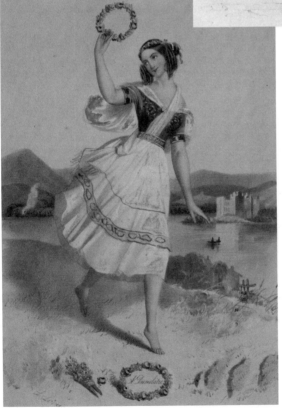

Adèle Dumilâtre in
Eucharis (choreography
by Coralli), 1844. Jerome
Robbins Dance Division;
New York Public Library
for the Performing Arts;
Astor, Lenox and Tilden
Foundations.

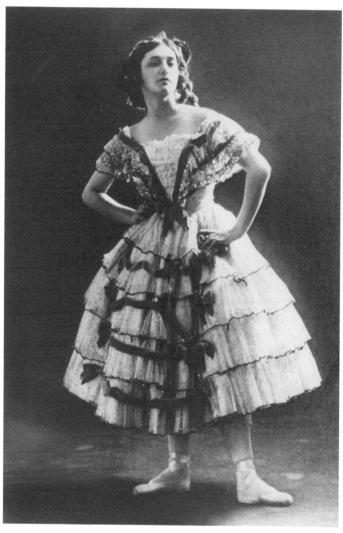

Tamara Karsavina in *Die Puppenfee*
(choreography by Hassreiter and Legat).
Jerome Robbins Dance Division; New
York Public Library for the Performing
Arts; Astor, Lenox and Tilden Foundations.

Tamara Karsavina in *La fille mal gardée* (choreography by Dauberval and Didelot). Jerome Robbins Dance Division; New York Public Library for the Performing Arts; Astor, Lenox and Tilden Foundations.

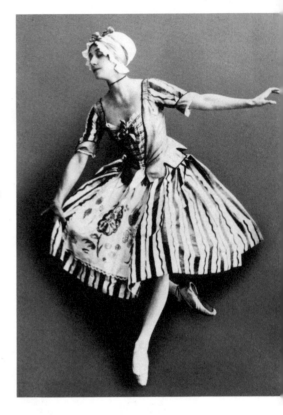

Tamara Karsavina in *Schéhérazade* (choreography by Fokine). Jerome Robbins Dance Division; New York Public Library for the Performing Arts; Astor, Lenox and Tilden Foundations.

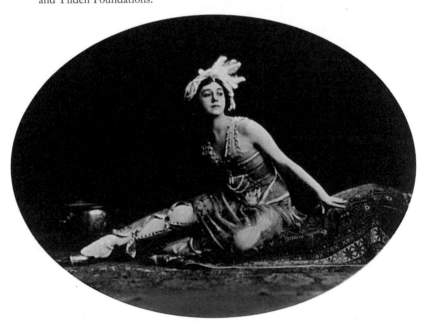

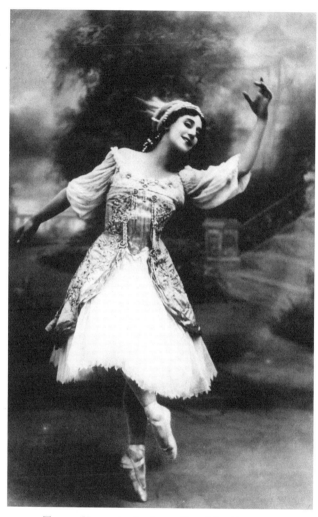

Tamara Karvsavina in *Le pavillon d'Armide*
(choreography by Fokine). Jerome Robbins
Dance Division; New York Public Library
for the Performing Arts; Astor, Lenox and
Tilden Foundations.

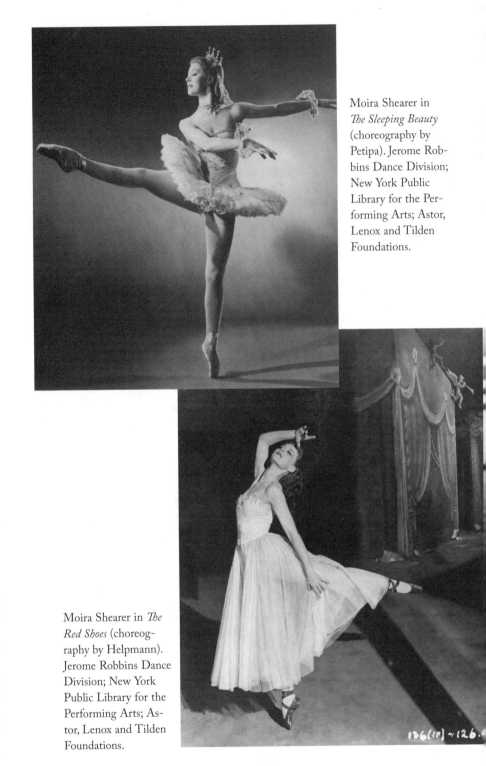

Moira Shearer in *The Sleeping Beauty* (choreography by Petipa). Jerome Robbins Dance Division; New York Public Library for the Performing Arts; Astor, Lenox and Tilden Foundations.

Moira Shearer in *The Red Shoes* (choreography by Helpmann). Jerome Robbins Dance Division; New York Public Library for the Performing Arts; Astor, Lenox and Tilden Foundations.

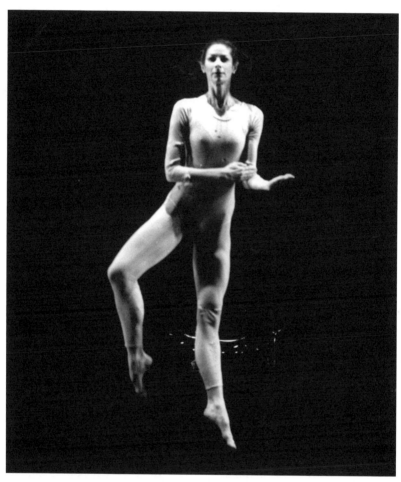

Catherine Kerr in *Rainforest*
(choreography by Cunningham),
1988. Courtesy Jed Downhill.

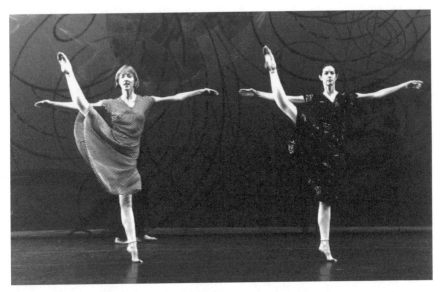

Catherine Kerr (right) with Victoria Finlayson
in *Fabrications* (choreography by Cunningham),
1987. Courtesy Jed Downhill.

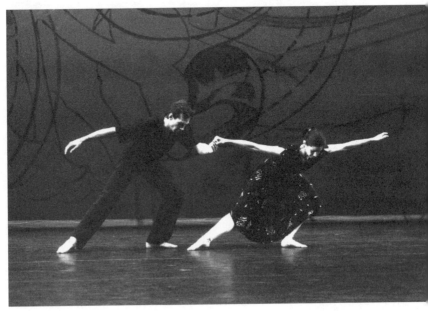

Catherine Kerr with Robert Swinston in
Fabrications (choreography by Cunningham),
1987. Courtesy Jed Downhill.

4

MOIRA
SHEARER

THE RED SHOES is a British movie produced and directed by Michael Powell and Emeric Pressburger in 1948. The screenplay was written by Pressburger; the film score, including the all-important music for a ballet within the film, was composed by Brian Easdale, and the choreography was by the renowned Australian dancer-actor Robert Helpmann. The beautiful Scottish-born ballerina Moira Shearer played the film ballerina Victoria (Vicky) Page. Anton Walbrook was the impresario Boris Lermontov; the famous real-life Russian choreographer Léonide Massine played the movie choreographer and ballet master; and Marius Goring was the brilliant, temperamental young composer, Julian Craster, who receives his first major commission to compose the score for the ballet. It is Julian who leads Vicky to abandon her profession for romance and marriage, and who ultimately drives the trapped and desperate young dancer to throw herself off a balcony in front of an onrushing train. In words that loom over Vicky's life and career, Lermontov describes Craster as embodying the "doubtful comforts of human love."

On one level, *The Red Shoes*, filmed in brilliant Technicolor, conforms to the pressure for realism that predominated in the 1940s British film industry; it avoids highly modernist tendencies, it demonstrates a coherent plot, and it achieves the twin goals of communication and entertainment. But as it operates within an ostensibly realistic vein, *The Red Shoes* also works at another level.

The director Martin Scorsese claims to have been drawn to the "hysteria" of the movie, which, according to the film scholar Ian Christie, subordinates narrative to an overriding sense of magic, exoticism, and larger-than-life passions. Christie maintains that audiences craved such surreal effects, for the movie "found a public more than ready to accept its fantasy and achieved a worldwide success, which continues to the present day."[1]

While Powell and Pressburger's film catered to a postwar audience craving kitsch, soap-opera romance, the directors simultaneously wove together elements of unarticulated myths and subconscious fantasies about the ballerina's noble dedication to her career. The film includes this exchange:

> Lermontov: Why do you want to dance?
> Vicky: Why do you want to live?
> Lermontov: I don't know exactly why, but I must.
> Vicky: That's my answer too.

As I read the movie's "message" today, I realize how confusing it is, and that its ending offers female dancers only the most narrow and bleak of options. The movie suggests that a female dancer must choose between career and family, that she must be glamorous and photogenic, and that her professional life demands an unreasonable degree of self-sacrifice. This grim message undercuts the heroine's red-haired, green-eyed screen loveliness, her precipitate escalation to fame, and her glamorous career against backdrops in London and Monte Carlo.

In fact, Moira Shearer's off-screen, real-life career was hardly less complicated than that depicted in the film. An acknowledged beauty, Shearer set about establishing herself as a professional ballet dancer during a devastating war; she emerged from wartime deprivations to appear in various films, and she married and started a family. In the midst of these early achievements, Shearer also confronted the iron will of Ninette de Valois, who, as director of the Vic-Wells Ballet, used her prerogative to promote Margot Fonteyn as the leading English ballerina.[2] Between them, the choreographer Frederick Ashton and Ninette de Valois primed Fonteyn to become a major English dancer, nurturing her development at the expense of other talented dancers like Shearer, Violetta Elvin, and Beryl Grey. Much like her screen character, Shearer may have felt the conflicts between her roles as artist, wife, and mother. She was notably dismayed over her lack of opportunities to create new ballets and to develop her artistry in the classics, a dismay that was shared by some dance writers of the day. I suspect that Shearer must have experienced personal turmoil and confusion as a young woman, and that early disappointments may have led her to retire prematurely from dance. Interviewers and dance writers who spoke with Shearer after her retirement have captured a sense of her disillusionment and her anxious perfectionism. It is this voice I hear today, as I go about filling in gaps in my understanding about Shearer's career and her sometimes uneasy relationship to life as a dancer.

Shearer called ballet a "selfish career," for once begun it must be pursued rigorously.[3] She would know: born Moira Shearer King in 1926 into an upper-middle-class family in Dunfermline, Scotland, she started ballet classes at age six in what was then Rhodesia. The classes were taught by a pupil of Cecchetti, Shearer recalled in a 1976 interview.[4] This teacher, Shearer said, "had been a proper dancer if I can put it like that. She really knew her stuff and she was Cecchetti trained." With parents and grandparents who were musical, Shearer found herself most drawn to music, but the ballet teacher encouraged her mother to continue Moira's ballet training when, two years later, the family relocated to London. Mrs. King was willing to give her daughter the finest training in the arts and took her to the studio of Nicolas Legat. In Shearer's words, "that was that." She remembers not having any communication with her mother regarding the classes. Her mother, she said, simply arranged things.[5]

Since the master did not train beginners, Shearer was first sent to Miss Flora Fairburn's classes, but when Fairburn took her to perform for Legat, the "heavenly old boy" accepted Moira immediately into his professional classes. After Legat's sudden death fifteen months later, Shearer continued her training with his wife. "I really did dislike it to begin with," Shearer told Barbara Newman. "As one hadn't chosen it for oneself, it was dismal to have to go through those tortures daily." But when she began to achieve a sense of mastery in the technique, her experience of dance changed and she found that she had begun to enjoy ballet class.[6]

When Britain was thrust into World War II, however, all normal life changed. Along with many other schools and ballet studios, the Legat school was evacuated, and the Sadler's Wells Theatre was taken over as a refuge for families made homeless in the air raids. Nonetheless, the gritty determination of Ninette de Valois, the theater's director, never wavered.[7] Even when the ballet company lost its premises and took to the road, touring the cities and provinces of England, the school continued to operate on the top floor of the Sadler's Wells Theatre, "in the large mirror-lined rehearsal room, with high glass windows," de Valois recalled. "Little King" as de Valois called her, was evacuated to the north with her family, but she would soon return to London and the Sadler's Wells "and blaze a trail as Moria Shearer."[8]

Later de Valois was able to describe this agonizing time in British history at a greater remove. At the time, however, and from the viewpoint of the young Moira Shearer, the evacuation and the unavoidable halt in training must have seemed endless. Without her ballet classes, in the midst of a terrifying air assault, "little King" was left rudderless; frustrated and depressed, she struggled to practice on her own. She was ready for the next step in her life. It came when, at age fourteen, she was invited to join Mona Inglesby's International Ballet. The year spent with Inglesby's ballet was both exciting and demanding, Shearer told *Ballet Today*. Her first exposure to theatrical life was complicated by the exigencies of performing and touring under wartime conditions, and she told of "standing in the wings while hasty last minute alterations were made to a dress she was wearing; and learning two new parts between matinee and evening performance."[9]

In 1942, when ballet performances resumed at the Sadler's Wells, Shearer left Inglesby and transferred to the Wells, where she was demoted to the *corps de ballet* and forced to give up the solo roles she had danced with the International Ballet. Shearer told Dale Harris that at Sadler's Wells she was required to take classes with the company for two weeks before she was allowed to join because "I came from—another company, my very first company which was the International Ballet. I had been for a year there. Because I was Russian trained which was frowned on then."[10] Her return to soloist was speedy, however, and eventually at the Wells she danced solos in Michel Fokine's *Les sylphides* and *Le spectre de la rose*, in Frederick Ashton's *Les patineurs*, and in Ninette de Valois's *The Gods Go a–Begging*. The following year she created the role of Pride in Ashton's *The Quest* (1943) and danced the *pas de trois* in de Valois's *Promenade* (1943).[11] In 1946 she was one of six dancers chosen by Ashton to originate roles in *Symphonic Variations*. As a ballerina, Shearer drew special attention from critics and audiences, dancing principal roles in *Coppélia, Swan Lake, Sleeping Beauty,* and *Giselle* and premiering the lead role (originally intended for Margot Fonteyn) in Ashton's *Cinderella* (1948).

During her career at the Wells, she occasionally accepted guest artist opportunities, leaving once to perform in Roland Petit's *Carmen* with his Ballets de Paris in 1950, once for the production of the *The Red Shoes,* and again for another film by Powell and Pressburger, the "daringly uncommercial" *Tales of Hoffman* (1950).[12]

As if her personal life were following the plot lines of the film she helped to popularize, Shearer stirred up controversy among her ballet colleagues when she married the writer Ludovic Kennedy in February 1950. The Wells dancers were curious at best about her decision. The ballerina Nadia Nerina recalls that at that point in the Sadler's Wells organization, "it was just unheard of" that a ballerina should marry. June Brae and Pamela May, both leading dancers with the Sadler's Wells, had been unable to manage the pressures of both careers and families and their professional lives began to peter out in spite of their best efforts. "I remember when Shearer got married," Nerina said. "All the eyebrows went flying high."[13]

Nevertheless, Shearer persisted in following her own goals; prior to the birth of her first daughter in 1952, she declared that she would combine the responsibilities of motherhood with her dance career. The *Evening Standard* for June 28, 1952, reported that she had been pondering her future as she awaited the birth of her child. If she was in any way undecided about her own plans, she was clear about her intentions for this unborn child. Both the *Daily Graphic* and the *Daily Sketch* for March 22, 1952, ran a photo of Shearer at practice. In the photo, she stands at the barre with her left leg bent into an attitude in the front, her left arm curved above her head; she wears a layered ballet skirt, and her ballet slipper has slipped off her raised foot. A caption apparently taken from Shearer announces "'MY CHILD WILL NOT BE A SLAVE'—SAYS BALLERINA." Both newspapers reported, "The red-haired 26 year-old dancing star gave her reasons last night in Hollywood, where she is making her first U.S. film. 'A ballet dancer must exercise, practise every day. You can never let down—if you do, you are finished.' Moira, who married author Ludovic Kennedy in February, 1950, began dancing at 10 and professionally at 15. Then the slavery began. . . . Having her child will mean her first holiday for 16 years, she says."

It must have seemed to Shearer and Kennedy that the press followed their every move. The *Star* (London) announced on May 2, 1952, "Moira is Home Again," after the dancer's return from the United States. The story noted, "Her red hair covered by a Paisley-style headscarf ballerina Moira Shearer, 26, who is expecting her first baby in August, reached Southampton today in the liner *Nieuw Amesterdam* from New York." Readers were also told that while she was in New York, Shearer had purchased a few baby items. The *Birmingham Gazette* for May 23, 1952, alerted readers to the intimate details: under a headline reading "Moira Shearer Back Home," the article reported, "'I'm hoping the baby will be a boy,' said the 26–year-old ballerina. 'I shall not be giving up my dancing career although at present I have no definite plans for the future.'" As it turned out, the baby was a red-haired girl and her weight was variously announced as 8 ½ or 8 ¼ pounds. On December 22, 1952, the *Star* ran a photo showing the couple on their way to a holiday in Copenhagen with their daughter, now five months old. Shearer, it was reported, was to "dance at Covent Garden next month."

As glamorous as any film star, Shearer found that in spite of herself she had become a public personality. In the *Evening Standard* (London) on May 1, 1953, in an article entitled "Beauty Begins at Home," James Mason's wife and Shearer offered beauty tips for busy women. Interested readers discovered that Moira Shearer "finds time between the 6 and 10 o'clock feed of baby Ailsa Margaret to wash, set and dry her hair. She tries to keep this time each day for her personal chores." The ballerina also gave pointers on waistline reduction exercises and ways to cut calories while still feeding the children properly. Shearer concluded by saying, "There would be fewer divorces if both men and women took a course on how to preserve glamour in the bedroom. If a wife is wise she finds time to make herself continually desirable."

For a time Shearer returned as a guest artist with the Sadler's Wells Ballet. It must have seemed an ideal plan: "She sees no reason why being a mother should prevent her from dancing. 'I know some people say it can't be done, but my home arrangements in Hampstead are perfect. I have a nanny and a housekeeper, so I can manage both the pram and the practice class.'"[14] But not long after fighting to regain her strength and technique following her maternity leave, Shearer decided to retire from dancing altogether. She was strained and fatigued, depleted by the increasing pressure to perfect herself and to compete with strong and brilliant rivals. She announced that she now hoped to devote herself to straight theater, cherishing the belief that an acting career would more easily accommodate her desires to spend time with her family. Peter Craig-Raymond, writing in *Ballet Today*, observed, "She is not the first artist who has had to choose between home and career, and, being a woman, it is not surprising that she has chosen the former: though in her case, of course, the choice was much less severe—it simply meant the abandoning of a successful career in ballet for the problematic one of the straight stage." Ballet makes demands, while an actor, Shearer explained with hopeful naivete, can be free during the day once a play is open. Further, when a dancer has achieved the status of ballerina, she must work ever harder to keep what she has gained because she can lose all her technique so quickly. Craig-Raymond reminisced about Shearer's career: "It is now nearly two years since she has danced at Covent Garden, and her place in the garland of ballerinas has never been filled, for she danced with a delicate, controlled beauty that was all her own, enchanting and enchanted."[15]

Did marriage and family seem the best, most reasonable life choice to a twenty-seven-year-old ballet dancer in 1953? After leaving dance, Shearer pursued a career in theater for five years. She then retired from the stage, though she appeared occasionally on radio and, later in her life, wrote reviews and a book entitled *Balletmaster: A Dancer's View of George Balanchine*. Nevertheless, in 1953, for the talented, glamorous, intelligent Moira Shearer, whose dance career started in 1940 at age fourteen, the future seemed to rest with her husband and children.

As noted earlier, Shearer's first instructor, in Ndola, Rhodesia, had trained in the Cecchetti method, a system introduced in the West when the Italian-born dancer and ballet master left his position at the Maryinsky Theatre to teach for the Diaghilev Ballets Russes. Upon assuming his post in Russia, Enrico Cecchetti brought to the Russian ballet the Italian training that prioritized technical virtuosity and strength; it was this emphasis on strength and technical precision that became codified in the Cecchetti teaching method.

During her childhood, Shearer experienced both the Cecchetti technique and the French-Russian training of Nicolas Legat. According to John Gregory and André Eglevsky, Legat studied with Cecchetti when the Italian maestro began teaching at the Imperial Theatre [Ballet] School in St. Petersburg. But, in contrast to what he learned from Cecchetti, Legat sought to preserve the "gracious 'French' style and the scientific yet creative freedom" acquired from another teacher at the Imperial Theatre School, the Swedish dancing master Christian Johannson (who also taught Mathilde Kchessinskya and Tamara Karsavina).[16] The Cecchetti and the Legat approaches to teaching were very different, and in all of her interviews Shearer identified herself as a product of Russian training.[17] She loved the Russian style, though the Italian school produced "a steely, brilliant technique which possibly the Russian style would never quite give you." But underneath it all, she registered her disapproval of the products of Cecchetti technique, of ballet taught as if it were a series of "stunts." "You go to the circus to see some fantastic thing on the trapeze, but it isn't beautiful; it's not what I feel the ballet should be about." And, she added, "I so much prefer the Russian style, and am so grateful that I had all my original training in that style."[18]

It was the Russian dancers, in the de Basil and the René Blum companies, who first shaped her notions about ballet. She recalled, "I was taken to Covent Garden when I was eight, and I remember the program exactly: it was *Sylphides, Boutique Fantasque* with Massine and Danilova, and *Contes Russes*."[19] Particularly impressive to the young Shearer were the dancers Vera Nemchinova and André Eglevsky.[20] She said, "I remember being most enamoured, crazy about

Eglevsky. All the dancers from these companies came to Legat's studio when they were in London and did classes with all of us. So as a small girl, one had the opportunity of watching these, to me, gods, which was a very great help for the future."[21]

Nicolas Legat's studio, with its stimulating mix of the finest European dancers, musicians, painters, and writers, proved a heady atmosphere for the young and talented dancer.[22] Shearer told Newman that, unlike the training she would later receive at de Valois's Sadler's Wells school, Legat's classroom exercises flowed like a real dance. "Everything," she said, "even at the barre, was arranged so that it gave you the impression of doing a little sequence of steps. Not quite a dance, but it was rounded off; you had a little ending." On the other hand, her experience of the Cecchetti training was that it was heavy, boring, and workmanlike. It was "bald," she explained, "eight of one step and puff and blow, turn around, and eight with the other leg, which was very much the case with British style. I found *those* classes an absolute torture because of it; there was no question of dancing at all, even when you came into the center."[23]

None of her later training at the Wells quite matched the experiences of those years with the Legats. Once she left the Legat studio and transferred to the Wells, she apparently felt bound by a stolid, codified rigidity. The training she received at the Wells was, for the most part, "terribly depressing." Shearer recalled that Ursula Moreton, "who'd been in Diaghilev's corps de ballet in the 1920s, gave a lot of classes, including special Cecchetti classes to which I said no firmly. I'd watched one or two of them through the glass door and thought, 'This is terrible. I don't want to do those.'" Moreton's approach, whether or not it was an accurate rendition of a Cecchetti class, was "totally mechanical," said Shearer. The Cecchetti training Shearer experienced focused only on the lower body, while Legat, true to his Russian-French lineage, emphasized the three-dimensional use of the back and the arms. "All that happened [in Cecchetti class] was from the waist to the tip of the foot, and nobody was bothering at all about what happened from the waist to the top of the head which, funnily enough, was the bit of one's body that Legat was much more interested in. . . . He was terribly anxious that your back and the carriage of your head were exactly right, and your arms and *épaulement*."[24]

Other Sadler's Wells teachers included Nicholas Sergeyev.[25] Shearer recalled him as "an enchanting old man, he couldn't have been nicer, but the classes he gave were terrible." She explained, "I just don't think he had the gift of teaching. He would do the worst things for one's leg muscles. He would give very slow développé at the barre, and then cause you to hold it for a very, very slow count of eight or ten. Then he would go 'round with his stick, hitting under the leg, harder than the dear old duck realized, to keep it up. In the end, the leg would just crash down; people would say, 'We can't take any more,' and he wouldn't really mind. But then you had to turn around and do it on the other side." While in Sergeyev's class, Shearer said, she knew that "this was harming one rather than helping," and that upon entering the daily class she usually felt "here is going to be a totally wasted hour and a quarter." Once in the company, her outlook did not improve, she said, as Ninette de Valois herself taught the company class: "And that was quite horrific in some ways, because she wasn't a natural teacher either. Everything was very busy and had to be done at twice the speed of light. She was a very fast, neat dancer herself and excelled in little batterie steps [small footwork, and quick jumps and beats], and people always do hone, quite unknowingly I think, to the way they dance themselves. It's inevitable. So her classes were pretty frenetic, one way or another, but not quite so damaging as old Sergeyev's."[26]

Even though Shearer complained about de Valois's quickness, she herself was also known for her lightness and her neat footwork, as Ashton's choreography in the first act of *Cinderella* (1948) would bear out. Julie Kavanaugh has called this ballerina's solo "a choreographic poem to Shearer's famously eloquent feet."[27] Although Shearer recalled feeling discomfort in de Valois's classes, her strain may well have been more emotional than physical.

In truth, the differences between Shearer and de Valois were not always great. While Shearer maintained that she preferred the French/Russian style to the "robot-like exercises" of the "British style" taught at the Wells, de Valois wrote that she too greatly valued the Russian training. In fact, de Valois had qualms about wholeheartedly adopting the Cecchetti method. She was well aware of her own diverse lineage and claimed to have drawn her pedagogical methods from a number of sources. De Valois (1898–2001) began her study with Cecchetti in 1919 while she was dancing with the Diaghilev Ballets Russes. Although she clearly admired Cecchetti's teaching, she was convinced that his "heavy" and "strength-building" method needed to be balanced by other approaches. "The many set exercises, heavy long *adagios* and systemised *enchainements,* in the end appear to be more rewarding for the male dancer than the female," she wrote.[28]

De Valois admired Legat's classes. As she attested, "From the beginning I could feel the deep knowledge behind the elegant but apparently free and easy approach, highlighted by the everlastingly new and very beautiful *enchainements* arranged from day to day." She believed that under Legat's tutelage she developed a new expansiveness and a fluid strength.[29] Other teachers of de Valois included Bronislava Nijinska, whose choreographic ideals and tendencies were "interwoven into our daily class."[30] Finally, de Valois added, she learned from the great Russian ballerina, Olga Preobrajenska, whose classes in her Paris studio were "most sound," and "devoid of any embellishments."[31] In de Valois's account, all these teachers influenced her own notions about training dancers and all contributed to what would become the British style. Without ambivalence, she labeled Shearer a product of the Sadler's Wells training: "by the outbreak of war," she wrote, the school had "produced Fonteyn, Brae, May, Grey, Shearer, Helpmann, Somes, Turner, Farron and others. All of them had a faithful audience who saw us into the Royal Opera House in 1946."[32]

But Shearer believed she was different from the other dancers at the Wells. And in some critical circles, she was described as not quite like the other British-trained dancers. The influence of her Russian training was perceptible to those who looked for it, and A. H. Franks, for one, referred to her as the auburn-haired, Russian-trained ballerina. Similarly, the impresario Sol Hurok reflected, "What impresses me most about Moira Shearer, the dancer, is a fluidity of movement that has about it a definite Russian quality; she has a fine polish in her style, coupled with great spontaneity and a gentle, easy grace."[33]

It was Marie Rambert and Ninette de Valois who were largely responsible for the availability of professional and pre-professional dance training in Britain and its colonies in the 1930s and the postwar era. The two women expended considerable devotion and energy to ensure that a native British ballet tradition would flourish where no consistent academic training had existed before.

Rambert (1888–1982) was born in Warsaw, Poland, and educated in the State School. Later she studied in Paris, where she became pupil and assistant to Jacques Dalcroze. In 1912 Dalcroze arranged to send her to Diaghilev to assist Vaslav Nijinsky in his choreography of Stravinsky's *Le sacre du printemps*. Though Rambert initially preferred Isadora Duncan's more free-flowing dance concerts to academic ballet, she found herself intrigued by the work she saw in the Diaghilev Ballets Russes.[34] She accepted Diaghilev's invitation to join the company and began her first formal ballet classes with Cecchetti. In the opinion of Alexander Bland, Rambert was "immensely energetic, musical, with an overpowering love of the theatre yet without great talent for dancing herself." Bland nonetheless believed that Rambert was "a born teacher."[35]

In 1920 Rambert opened a school in London and within six years organized a concert by her students at the Lyric Theatre, Hammersmith. Among these first students was the young choreographer Frederick Ashton, whose early promise Rambert was to nurture and develop. The list of her homegrown British students is impressive; it included Antony Tudor, Andrée Howard, Pearl Argyle, and Maude Lloyd. With her husband, the British playwright Ashley Dukes, Rambert bought a church hall in Ladbroke Road and turned it into a studio and showcase for her little company.

Bland says that Rambert had precisely the temperament to permit such a venture to succeed on a minimal budget. Rambert displayed, he said, "an obsessional and fanatical concentration on her work; a ferocious continental personality which expressed itself, now in raptures, now in screams and tantrums; an uncanny eye for detail, whether it was a misplaced finger, a faulty shoulder-strap or a sixpence squandered on a bit of ribbon." She brought these evenings of ballet to fruition as she "drove, cajoled, tricked and magnetised" her students "into enthusiastic and self-sacrificing collaboration. Hard as she worked everybody, she spared no one less than herself."[36] Eventually, however, many of her students would leave her for Ninette de Valois and the greater opportunities she offered. Rambert trained, fostered, and encouraged her pupils and then witnessed the flowering of Britain's first generation of entirely homegrown ballet dancers and choreographers, mainly at de Valois's Sadler's Wells company.

When the Irish-born Ninette de Valois (born Edris Stannus) began her training in London, she was first sent to Mrs. Wordsworth's Edwardian School of Deportment. In line with the mores of polite society in the breaking years of the twentieth century, Wordsworth's instruction was aloof from any odor of "professionalism." Wordsworth had it in her mind that hers was a school for young ladies, and she taught them a genre called "fancy dancing," which, said de Valois, "was harmless and good fun." Wordsworth had "a puritanical loathing of dancing as a profession" and demanded that her pupils "eschew the theatrical profession at all costs." De Valois concluded, "I wasted valuable years as a Wordsworth show pupil displaying a pair of painfully untheatrical feet."[37]

Recognizing that her daughter was an unusually talented dancer, de Valois's mother made a disruptive break with Mrs. Wordsworth and sent the teenager to the Lila Field Academy, which de Valois recalled as "a typical theatrical school. We learnt something of everything, but I was almost immediately set aside to specialize in the classical ballet section." In 1913, the fourteen-year-old de Valois was one of a group of students sent on tour—as the Wonder Children—to perform a series of short ballets and plays. Each of the Wonder Children represented one of the "great stars." "Needless to say," she writes, "I was doomed to be Pavlova and executed The Dying Swan, having laboriously noted this down myself from the upper circle of the Palace Theatre."[38]

The dance enthusiast A. H. Franks has decribed the state of dance education and appreciation in Britain at the beginning of the twentieth century:

> In England the situation was desperate, for this country had no real company of its own. As is so typical of the English character—which sees in ourselves a sort of general superiority over all other races, but a definite inferiority in each particular art and science—our critics saw very little possibility of the development of native talent. Indeed, some of the more cynical and stupid of them openly asserted that the Russian Ballet was so much a product of Russia that it was absurd for us to attempt to produce what must ever remain nothing but a travesty of Russian achievement.[39]

De Valois was to commit much of her energy, devotion, and commanding presence to correcting the deficit in training and, simultaneously, to rectifying this national inferiority complex. For her, it was the lack of training standards that held British dancers back from achieving true excellence, just as it was the devaluing of dance as a theatrical art that prevented the flourishing of ballet in general. In the course of her long career at the Royal Ballet, the zealous de Valois permitted Britain's choreographers to test their wings; nudged, provoked, prodded, and fostered her dancers; shaped the taste and trained the eyes of her audiences; and founded a national ballet company. But de Valois recognized her indebtedness to others, noting that the birth of a ballet tradition in Britain depended on those gifted artists who were uprooted from their own native countries through war and revolution. "It is hard to imagine what would have influenced the English and American Schools of Ballet had it not been for the 1914 war and the Russian Revolution," she wrote.[40] De Valois freely acknowledged that her work with the Diaghilev Ballets Russes was a source of personal inspiration while it also served to stimulate a larger public appetite for dance. It was the Diaghilev Ballets Russes and its successors—among them the Ballet Russe de Monte Carlo and the de Basil Ballet Russe—that began to build audiences for dance throughout dance-starved regions of western Europe and America.

Further, it was her experiences as a dancer in Diaghilev's company (1923–25), de Valois later explained, that introduced her to the notion of professionalism in dance. As she mingled with displaced Russian artists who arrived in the West, trailing the remnants of their Imperial Ballet traditions, de Valois came to see dancers as dedicated professionals striving for excellence. Her years with the great Russian dancers led her to realize that dancers in a ballet company must live according to a "rigid code of discipline and community life carried to fantastic lengths."[41] She was hence determined on her course: to create a

British ballet tradition she must establish a company that operated on just such high standards of artistic creation and disciplined training.

Once her plan was laid, de Valois pursued it determinedly. Kathrine Sorley Walker describes some of de Valois's ideas, which she had begun to formulate as early as 1930: "Looking ahead, she knew that as time went on she would need various elements for developing her little ballet group into a strong and important company. Another choreographer besides herself, a prima ballerina and *premier danseur,* an able musical director and conductor. From what she had seen of his work [Frederick] Ashton seemed to her the best choice as choreographer."[42]

De Valois strategically plotted her course in building the company she envisioned, her goal being to bring fine ballet, including both classical and new works, to the British public. She moved decisively toward this goal, inevitably sacrificing some talented dancers in order to nurture others. According to David Vaughan, de Valois recognized that the brilliant young British choreographer Antony Tudor would one day develop into a creative genius, but he was not the classical choreographer she sought. Ashton was. And it was Margot Fonteyn she chose to develop as company ballerina after Alicia Markova's departure, though younger gifted dancers—Beryl Grey and Moira Shearer among them—waited eagerly for new challenges.[43]

There are a number of reasons why these challenges were never forthcoming for Shearer, as they would be for Fonteyn. One reason was the movie. Shearer's decision to appear in *The Red Shoes* was not an easy one, nor was it made quickly; she had to be pushed to accept Michael Powell's offer of a starring role.[44] From the beginning, she says, she had disliked the script and story, which she found untrue to real-life ballet companies. But, after much pestering from Powell, she was advised by Ninette de Valois to accept his offer. De Valois reportedly told her, "For heaven's sake, child, get this off your chest, *and* ours, because I can't stand these men bothering all of us any longer."[45] In succumbing to Powell's pressure, though, Shearer found herself in a tangle of unpleasantness. Not only was de Valois convinced that all ballet on film was a "vulgarity," Daneman writes, she managed to convey to Shearer that "most people in highbrow artistic circles considered a film contract to be little better than a pact with the devil."[46]

In time, the consequences of her film appearance became clear to Shearer, for "the ballet purist resented the fact that she had made a film at all," while the "film world was aggrieved because she had criticised methods of film technique as applied to ballet, and because she refused to make another film."[47] The media attention she garnered was virtually unprecedented in the dance world, and the glitzy quality of Hollywood publicity did not sit well with de Valois, who had worked to establish ballet as a serious art form. Shearer "was now subjected to a glare of publicity, unlike anything experienced in ballet, often embarrassing and ruthless and from which she was never to be entirely free. She said she began to dread picking up a newspaper in case she found herself misrepresented or the centre of some controversy."[48]

Nevertheless, Shearer's role in *The Red Shoes* was significant in helping to shape twentieth-century European and American attitudes toward ballet. Despite its melodrama, *The Red Shoes* marked a sea change in its depiction of the female ballet dancer, as Vicky Page is no courtesan or ballet girl dependent on a wealthy lover for protection and support. The ballet world imagined in the Powell-Pressburger film is one of heightened reality and tempestuous emotions where ballerinas live and die for their art. In the world established by *The Red Shoes*, ballet stars exist in passionate celibacy; they are glamorous, photogenic creatures who wear modish clothes and travel to sun-drenched Mediterranean locales to perform for audiences composed of intellectuals, artists, and members of high society. The good ones—the most highly talented ballerinas (these demands are never apparently placed on male dancers)—tear themselves away from lives of potential ease and domestic happiness. At the opening of the film we learn that Vicky Page is no run-of-the-mill young lady. An heiress, she comes from a wealthy family of socialites; viewers are asked to sympathize with how much she has given up in order to develop her talents as a dancer.

The mixed messages of the film coexist uneasily. In some sense, the ballet dancers in *The Red Shoes* have all the popularly imagined characteristics of movie stars: they are beautiful, public, and dramatic figures. But they are unlike movie idols in their highly disciplined, humble, and self-sacrificing approaches to their work. As she appeared to embody all these fantasies, Moira Shearer won the hearts of millions of viewers. While the making of the film was distasteful for Shearer and its eventual impact on her career may have been detrimental, *The Red Shoes* was an enormous popular success and introduced vast numbers of middle-class movie-goers to a world of ballet they would otherwise not have known.[49]

Once the film came out, Shearer was besieged by fans and, as Meredith Daneman puts it, "A vast new international audience of filmgoers now knew of only one English ballerina. And her name was not Margot Fonteyn."[50] Plenty of Americans, for instance, who had been riveted by Shearer's performance in the film, looked forward to her 1949 visit to the United States, though they may have been only vaguely impressed that she would be accompanied by the Sadler's Wells Ballet Company. The *New York Herald Tribune* for October 16, 1949, previewed the "Dancing Visitors from Abroad," with a photograph of—not Margot Fonteyn—but the second-tier ballerina Moira Shearer in her costume for the title role in Ashton's *Cinderella*. On October 17, 1949, in the same newspaper, it was reported that *The Red Shoes* had completed a successful yearlong run in New York's Bijou cinema. A popular American women's magazine ran a photo of Shearer, dressed in practice clothes, leaning against a wall, as if at rest from rehearsal. The caption reads, "Moira Shearer, the exquisite young star of the ballet film *The Red Shoes*, comes to America this month with British Sadler's Wells Ballet. The company of sixty, with incomparable Margot Fonteyn as prima ballerina, will tour the United States and Canada after a four-week engagement at the Metropolitan Opera House."[51]

The dance critic Clive Barnes claimed that de Valois banked on Shearer's popularity to entice American audiences to the Metropolitan Opera House on the occasion of the company's first New York tour, in 1949. In Barnes's telling of the story, Moira Shearer was an opening act for Margot Fonteyn.[52] American audiences would be lured to the Met by Shearer, de Valois believed, but they would stay to see Fonteyn and the Sadler's Wells Ballet. Nadia Nerina supported Barnes's version of events. Sol Hurok produced the company's tour, Nerina said, only "because of *The Red Shoes*." Nerina remarked, "Otherwise Hurok wouldn't have taken the company. Pamela May, Margot Fonteyn—who knew *them* in America?" American audiences did know Shearer, though, and Hurok advocated that the opening night in New York should be given to Shearer.[53]

De Valois won her point that Margot Fonteyn should have the starring role in *The Sleeping Beauty* on opening night but agreed that Moira Shearer would appear in a less-important role. Shearer told Daneman that she had assumed she would dance her familiar roles in *The Sleeping Beauty*, the Fairy of the Crystal Fountain (act 1) and one of Florestan's sisters (act 3).[54] Instead, she said, "Ninette did something bad to me at the beginning of the season so that I would go down the drain, and I was just too confused not to do what she asked."[55] Unexpectedly, de Valois told her she would dance the Bluebird *pas de deux* in the third act of the ballet with Alexis Rassine. Shearer recalled,

> I never was absolutely certain if I could produce all the technical fireworks again and again, and the nerve strain was very great. De Valois knew this absolutely. And with the Bluebird, I had until the third act that night and she knew I would get in way before the performance began and put my make-up on, and warm up and do my class. But I would have to sit through the whole

evening in the dressing room and I would be a wreck by the time it got to the Bluebird. She was absolutely right! She couldn't have been more right. The silly thing was that almost everybody else in the company seem to have been aware of this and thought me a perfect fool not to have refused this arrangement but I just didn't think you *could* refuse. I was very naive I suppose but I never did say, "No I won't do anything," or "I want to do something." I just felt one didn't do that.[56]

Nerina told Daneman that Shearer could have refused de Valois but didn't. "They were all so petrified of Ninette," she said. "Moira only had to say 'No I'm not doing it, I'll wait until I appear as Princess Aurora.' . . . One can only speculate on what effect a Shearer first night would have had on Margot's career, and whether Moira herself realizes, to this day, the enormity of the error she made."[57]

Violetta Elvin, Shearer's Russian-born friend and frequent dressing-room companion, concurred that the "problem" for Shearer hinged on *The Red Shoes:* "In Moira's career, her luck of *Red Shoes,* it was her ruin as a ballerina. It turned so many people against her because she suddenly jumped to stardom, slightly round-ways, which is not sometimes appreciated in a big organization."[58] Elvin described the conflict as "tremendous trouble with Moira and Margot because in America everybody wanted to see Moria Shearer because of *The Red Shoes.* That's why I was mentioning how really Moira ruined her career *in* the company because of *Red Shoes.*" Elvin suggested that Shearer's stardom antagonized various factions of the company. She had "overjumped" and become "more powerful than they wished her to be." In other countries, Elvin declared, a dancer's talent wins out, "but in England, you wait your turn."[59] Indeed, Shearer's own sense of "differentness" from the others trained at the Wells operated against what Alistair Macaulay has dubbed the "Vic-Wells sense of personal subordination to a larger cause."[60] As director of the Sadler's Well Ballet, de Valois considered it her duty to position herself as a pragmatic and somewhat ruthless leader; if Shearer suffered casualties in this event, it was, in the long run, all for the betterment of the company.

According to Daneman, though, antagonism toward Shearer came not only from de Valois, and it was not motivated simply by jealousy over her film success. Other Wells dancers resented that she had "overjumped," and Shearer's shyness was often taken for aloofness (according to her husband). Her reserve had made her unpopular with the *corps de ballet,* while Fonteyn was well liked by her colleagues, who thought she was charming, sweet tempered, and professional.[61]

Evidence of Fonteyn's own sense of the rivalry came to light with the publication of her autobiography. In 1976 Fonteyn was bitingly honest in discussing her perception that Shearer might jeopardize her prominence as prima ballerina. The experience of stepping aside to allow Shearer to dance the lead in *Cinderella* was more profound than many people realized. Fonteyn writes,

> I had risen to the top while very young, and now I had to concern myself with staying there. This is much the hardest aspect of success.... I simply had not thought about the dancers coming up from behind, and likely to overtake me. Beryl Grey was a lot younger than I and easily fitted her place as a ballerina, sharing the classical roles. Violetta Elvin brought new life from her Russian background and so gave more than she took. Then came Moira Shearer, with her incredible airy lightness and ease, to be a real threat to my position. Moira was young, fresh, beautiful and different.[62]

At one point during the company's rail tour of the United States and Canada, Shearer was "moved up" to share both dressing room and train sleeping compartment with Fonteyn. Fonteyn's usual dressing-room partner, Pamela May, had flown home with a knee cartilage problem and "it was a question of who would go in with Margot." Shearer was horrified, she said, to find her name go up: "nobody said anything to me—you just saw it on the board." The two ballerinas had coexisted for years without having a conversation, said Shearer. She admitted to finding it difficult to talk with Fonteyn, who could be "enigmatic to the point of being quite chilly sometimes." After a short time sharing quarters, Shearer realized that Fonteyn might well be the more nervous of the two. Shearer then decided to "be myself, and try and make her laugh.... by the end of those months she was a totally different person—she even swore, once or twice, quite strongly, and I thought, my goodness, she's really loosened up."[63]

No matter what competition might have existed between the two women, Shearer considered herself lucky never to be one of de Valois's favorites.

> Now, I think this is important to say. Sooner or later, particular people come along who the director particularly likes. It's not absolute favoritism, but it does happen ... in all companies probably.... it's only human. There were one or two, of my age or slightly older, who went through a phase of this, or de Valois went through a phase on them so to speak. To my great good luck, she never had any phase on me at all, which I found a very good thing. Too much would be given to the dancer of the moment, and nobody could ever fulfill all that was expected, whereupon they would be dropped.[64]

Still, the idea that Shearer was bypassed in favor of Fonteyn has been iterated by a number of people familiar with the inner workings of the Sadler's Wells.[65] Elvin said she found it difficult to forgive her contemporaries for neglecting Shearer's special gifts.

> She was such a talented person and so beautiful, so ethereal, fragile to give an impression from the public. And the quality that she had was sometimes criticized by people that maybe didn't realize that this is her. They criticize her for her quality of being as if slightly cold and brisk. But that was Moira. If she stayed in our company . . . with Sadler's Wells where they knew her, I'm sure, if she would be patient, Frederick Ashton, Macmillan, and other choreographers of the company would have written ballets specially for her which nobody could have copied because it would have been her, her "place" [French pronunciation] . . . and she would have stood up and would have had a lot of satisfaction.[66]

Shearer later spoke openly of experiencing what must have felt like an almost pathological anxiety.

> I think, looking back, I was temperamentally unsuited to be in the ballet. I don't think it was really my thing in the way Spessivtzeva, for instance, was obviously unsuited temperamentally and it was too much of a strain. In a totally different, very lesser way, I think I had the same problem because I suffered from the most terrible nerves you can imagine. I tried not to let this show through too much but I used to go through agonies before performances especially over the big classics because I was never a great thundering technician.[67]

The strain that Shearer felt in striving to satisfy herself, her colleagues, de Valois, and those dance critics who invariably compared her to Fonteyn may well have seemed unbearable for a talented young woman in her midtwenties. Among other qualities, critics frequently commented on the women's physical differences: Fonteyn, with her large dark eyes, dark hair and pale skin, could appear exotic, dramatic, warm. Shearer's porcelain delicacy, on the other hand, was sometimes described as detrimental to her stage presence. According to some commentators, Shearer's appearance of fragility and her burst of red hair made her a striking beauty on film but meant she was incapable of projecting across what then seemed to be the vast space at the Covent Garden Opera House, where the ballet company moved at the conclusion of World War II.[68] Unlike Fonteyn, Shearer could never be the "foremost British ballerina."

Indeed, looks dictated much of Shearer's career. In large part because of her physical appearance, she found that she was often cast as Swanilda in *Cop-*

pélia, a bright, mischievous soubrette role that many felt suited her coloring and her light quickness as a dancer. But, Shearer said, "I never enjoyed [it] at all, and unfortunately was always hideously successful" in the role. "I found it arch and pert, all the things I really don't like, and terribly mock-jokey in the middle act." She demurred slightly, "One was very lucky to be doing it at all, I suppose, but I could well have done without it occasionally."[69]

Nevertheless, Shearer did have the opportunity to test her wings in other cherished ballerina roles. She talked to Newman about her memories of dancing *The Sleeping Beauty:* "I adored doing the Rose Adagio, but I had kittens, right 'til the very last time I ever danced Aurora, over the variation that follows it. If you break it down into the actual steps, there's nothing so very difficult in it, yet I was so nerve-wracked over it that I never once did it perfectly."[70]

When Shearer made her debut in *The Sleeping Beauty*, the critics fell into two camps: those who hoped to see her develop in the role, and those who ranked her as inferior to Fonteyn. In his review of the 1946 season, Arnold Haskell registered his "surprise" at Shearer's successful *Sleeping Beauty*. He was decidedly ambivalent, however, for he was taken aback by her "un-Britishness" and her refusal to apologize or hesitate. He remarked on her "attack and a self-possession altogether unusual in a young British dancer." She won the audience over from the moment she appeared, wrote Haskell. "Never was a dancer less apologetic for any errors of technique, with the result that technical shortcomings due to inexperience are not noticed." She made a false entrance, which she covered with "aplomb." And he granted that she had "a magnificently fluid style, great and unusual beauty and a fine intelligence." He looked forward to a year hence when "her technique has caught up with her very conscious artistry, she should become an outstanding member of the company. She is in the potential ballerina class."[71]

Later, writing in the *Illustrated Magazine* of November 2, 1946, Haskell described the "young titian-haired dancer" as having caused a "balletic sensation" at her debut performance of *The Sleeping Beauty*. "Her beauty may have been an advantage in focusing the public attention," Haskell said, but "it could also have been a handicap to her artistic career had she lacked the ability to exploit it properly." Haskell predicted that "in Moira Shearer our national ballet has found a dancer of international status." Only an expert, he hinted, could see signs of nervousness in the slight strain of her mouth.

In June 1946, Audrey Williamson noted the exceptional position of Margot Fonteyn as the leading English ballerina: "It is, moreover, doubtful if any country in the world to-day can show a Princess Aurora of greater artistic completeness, more apparent ease of execution and range of poetic expression, than that of Margot Fonteyn." But one of the other fine performances that season was Moira Shearer's Aurora. Her lack of experience with the role "meant an occasional awkwardness of transition from position to position; but her balance, carriage and high arabesque line, and her swift precision of technique, mark her as a ballerina with a brilliant future."[72]

Mary Clarke, writing of the first postwar season of Sadler's Wells, in 1945–46, had a different take on Shearer's performance. She believed Shearer's first Aurora was "a little superficial from the dancing point of view, but extraordinarily mature as a piece of stage craft." Clarke remarked that Shearer looked exquisite, though "the very delicacy and fragility of her style robbed it of effectiveness when seen from a great distance, and throughout her career at Covent Garden she remained a dancer for the stalls rather than for the amphitheatre or gallery."[73]

Even beyond her film star popularity, Shearer did have substantial success dancing leading roles in New York. In the *New York Times* on September 16, 1950, John Martin described a more mature performance by Shearer: "Though the Sadler's Wells Ballet has been dancing at the Metropolitan Opera House for the better part of a week, it was not until last night that Moira Shearer, one of its major artists, made her first appearance. It was an event eminently worth waiting for, however, for Miss Shearer is dancing like a dream." Shearer made a "winning" Princess, wrote Martin, "charming to look at, dainty, precise, and full of spirit." Martin was clearly impressed with her virtuosity as well: "Technically she is prodigious," for Shearer, he continued, "tosses off the 'Rose Adagio' with ease and aplomb, and exhibits a marvelous brilliance in the several variations. She has an exceptional ability to put over a bravura passage for all it is worth, without being in the least aggressive about it or forfeiting anything whatever of its artistic values."

While Martin claimed that "Miss Shearer garbs her bravura in the most delightful modesty," Walter Terry, writing in the *New York Herald Tribune* on October 16, 1949, was not quite as impressed. "There were times," he noted, "when the ballerina concluded a virtuosic phrase or a dance with some rather heavy flourishes. Flourishes are, of course, permissible and our own American dancers are certainly given to circusy finales, but Miss Shearer's dancing was distinguished by such dignity that closing flourishes provided unexpected jolts." Terry made no bones about his preference for Fonteyn: "This charming and proficient dancer, known to American audiences through her motion picture, *The Red Shoes,* cannot hope to rival the company's prima ballerina, Margot Fonteyn, in this demanding assignment, but she does give a performance which is very much worth seeing."

Shearer was "regal," said Terry, and "mature rather than girlish." Though she danced with precision and style, "she does not always sustain the quality of lyricism throughout a movement sequence, but a wonderful mobility in the shoulders and back enables her to capture this necessary motor quality on those occasions when movement patterns are allocated to those portions of the body." Terry closed with a tribute: "In the main, however, Miss Shearer's performance was one worthy of a young ballerina and a very beautiful ballerina at that."

A rare opportunity to create the leading role in the first full-evening ballet created by a British choreographer came Shearer's way in 1948. Frederick Ashton's three-act *Cinderella*, to the score by Serge Prokofiev, was a significant pioneering effort for the Sadler's Wells Ballet, and a major role for Shearer. Fonteyn had been Ashton's choice for the role of Cinderella, but she had torn a ligament on the opening night of his one-act *Don Juan*. Thus, the new full-length ballet opened on Christmas Eve 1948 with Moira Shearer in the leading role. Cinderella was a role that, for the most part, was built around Moira Shearer, as David Vaughan explains:

> Ashton says that he had done hardly any work with Fonteyn herself on the longer ballet before her injury. So that it was Shearer who, he says in a revealing phrase, "dragged it out of me," and the role was clearly made to exploit her best features, the brilliance of her technique and her lightness. Many people have said that only when Fonteyn finally appeared in the ballet (which did not happen until 25 February 1949) did the character come fully to life. Undoubtedly she was, then and for many years afterwards, its ideal interpreter, but Ashton says that he was very pleased with Shearer, that she was an underrated dancer, perhaps because of her great personal beauty. But it was left to Fonteyn to fulfil the pathos of the character.[74]

Some of the critics warmed to Shearer in this role, though it was everywhere made apparent that the part rightfully belonged to Fonteyn. With Fonteyn's injury, observed Mary Clarke, the part of Cinderella was "entrusted to Moria Shearer, then at the height of her *Red Shoes* film fame." Shearer confronted the challenge, rising "to it without betraying any sign of nervousness. Looking lovely and elegant as any film star among the cinders, she danced with a new-found freedom and swiftness, and in the beautiful ballroom *pas de deux* she showed feeling as well."[75]

In his music for the ballet, Prokofiev sought to explore the blossoming of Cinderella's love, the obstacles confronting her, and then the fulfillment of this ideal love. While the poetic story appealed to Ashton and matched his choreographic interests, in the long run, many viewers have come to feel that the production is instead dominated by the broad characterizations of the stepsisters, originally danced *en travestie* by Helpmann and Ashton himself. Walter Terry, reviewing the first New York performances of the ballet in the *Herald Tribune* of October 20, 1949, certainly thought the production was unbalanced. He noted that the stage picture was overtaken by the clowning of Helpmann and Ashton. The ballet "belongs to them," wrote Terry. "Miss Shearer, in the peculiar position of a star with a minor role, helps wherever possible in making *Cinderella* seem (and Miss Fonteyn worked a similar bit of magic) much better than it actually is." While continuing to measure Shearer against Fonteyn, Terry found much to applaud in Shearer's performance. Her characterization was "winning" and her performance clear and precise. And, while it "seems to be Miss Shearer's lot to follow Margot Fonteyn," in this case the second ballerina held her own:

> Perhaps the pure dance passages are not quite as lyrical as those offered by Miss Fonteyn, but the dramatic shadings of the part are more varied in color and more penetrating in Miss Shearer's presentation. At the hearthside, she is more than wistful. She is broken-hearted, she is shyly defiant, she finds delicious hope in reverie. These tumbling emotional states are clearly projected by Miss Shearer at the opening of the ballet, and later, as the toast of the Prince's fete, she is more joyous (although it is a reserved and well bred sort of joy) in spirit than is Fonteyn in this same scene.

In his *Symphonic Variations,* a 1946 work of "pure dance," Ashton deployed six dancers as "equals" on the stage to create what many considered a sparse and "abstract," highly musical masterpiece of twentieth-century British ballet. Ashton chose to use the ballerinas Fonteyn, Shearer, and Pamela May with their partners, Michael Somes, Henry Danton, and Brian Shaw, as a unified ensemble. To music by César Franck and with decor and costumes by Sophie Fedorovich, the work "expressed the metaphysical thoughts that had fascinated him during the war," Alistair Macaulay wrote.[76] Hurok described the ballet's appeal for him: it was a work utilizing "three couples, on an immense stage in an immensely effective setting of great simplicity by Sophie Fedorovich." There was "no virtuoso role," and it comes across as "a lyric work, calm, ordered, in which the classical spirit is exalted in a mood of all for one, one for all."[77] De Valois called the ballet "one of our major successes." She noted its "abstract simplicity" and "lineal purity." A true ensemble work, "it spoke boldly from the huge stage," and the dancers filled the "space with the speed of meteors; here was a study in neo-classicism of the highest quality."[78] Writing in the *Nation* of the ballet's first New York performance, B. H. Haggin had a relatively favorable initial response.[79] On October 29, 1949, he noted particularly the "exquisite quiet elegance" of Margot Fonteyn as well as Brian Shaw's virtuosity and "good manners."[80]

In spite of its atmosphere of elegance and serenity, *Symphonic Variations* was a marathon for all involved, Margaret Dale told David Vaughan. Clearly, the ensemble had been well chosen, for the ballet made demands in terms of stamina and performance integrity. Vaughan wrote,

> It was a test of sheer stamina that very few British dancers could stand at that time. . . . The original cast rose magnificently to the occasion. Fonteyn remains incomparable—her stamina at least was never in question after all the gruelling years of touring, and her performance established her once and for all as the exemplar of the national style that Ashton was beginning to create. The fair Pamela May and the red-headed Moira Shearer, who had both danced Aurora in the new *Beauty*, were the obvious, perfect complements to Fonteyn, and her equals in the purity of their classicism.[81]

Mary Clarke called the ballet "a shaft of sunshine" and "perhaps the most completely beautiful dance composition Sadler's Wells had ever presented." There was no virtuoso dancing here, she wrote, nothing to draw one's attention to one dancer over another. Instead, "it was unceasingly lovely and created an impression of effortless lyricism and almost godlike serenity which at moments quickened under the urgent tempo of the music." She commended all the performers for enabling the choreographer to realize his intentions. They gave their utmost to fulfill "the design of the ballet as a whole and none [tried] to obtrude their own personalities."[82]

While *Symphonic Variations* was noted as a critical success as well as a "marathon" for the dancers, Shearer was unfazed by its demands and by its success. She recognized that her role in this abstract ballet was to serve the overall stage design:

> *Symphonic Variations* is simply steps, pure dancing. There isn't anything else for the public to hang onto; but that, surely, is what you learn to do as a dancer. You are simply there in *Symphonic*, on a stage, and you have to try to create a series of geometric patterns, to music, that are genuinely beautiful to look at. And create some kind of illusion or mood of . . . coolness or excitement. That's why it's terribly important to have exactly the right scenery and costumes, because the mood and atmosphere of those abstract ballets are all-important.[83]

Although she spoke fondly of several ballets, without hesitation Shearer identified *Giselle* as her most cherished role. "I had always wanted to do *Giselle*, always," she told Newman. Inevitably, though, she found Fonteyn's performance was "stamped on that production, and you were just put into it." It was difficult for her to make the role her own. So, on her own initiative, Shearer contacted Tamara Karsavina, "which got me into a certain amount of trouble at the time but paid off in the end." Really, said Shearer, it was "madness not to get in touch with this woman," who lived in London and remembered how "this was danced at the Maryinsky and who has danced it herself many times."[84]

Karsavina welcomed the invitation to coach Shearer. The younger woman recalled that "when I arrived, I just plunged straight in, and the dear old thing had the rug back and was demonstrating for me." The two discussed staple elements of the Sadler's Wells production that did not ring true for Shearer. Some of the mimed passages Karsavina demonstrated seemed more believable to the character Shearer was working on developing, "like the way Giselle moves forward when she encounters Bathilde and sees the court clothes for the first time. In our production, it was just, 'Isn't it lovely?' The way Karsavina showed it was both less kittenish and less arch than that. She did it with absolute amazement, as if being drawn forward, not wanting to go at all. In fact, the movements can be almost the same, but if you have that attitude and try to get that across the vista to the people out there, it has a quite different effect."[85]

In the end, Shearer said, she was able to incorporate only some of Karsavina's coaching suggestions, but when de Valois saw these details for the first time at Shearer's matinee performance, she stormed backstage to the dressing room. Shearer remembered,

> Although I'd done only minute things, she was absolutely furious and thought that this was just my own idea. The temerity of someone my age to do this! She really bawled me out—and I had got the second act coming up, and I'd never danced it before. Then she said, in the general tirade, Who did I think I was? What did I think I was doing? and Where had I got these ludicrous ideas anyway? So I just said, "Anything that you find unacceptable I got from Madame Karsavina, whom I went to see because I was interested enough to find out her view of the part."[86]

No doubt the challenge to her authority took de Valois by surprise: "That stopped her absolutely cold," said Shearer. "And the next thing I knew, Karsavina had been invited for special rehearsals with Margot and whoever she was dancing with at the time."[87] In the final analysis, said Shearer, she believed the overall production was improved, but she regretted that the rest of the company was not invited to the coaching sessions with Karsavina. "Wasn't it odd? Wouldn't it have been fascinating for the whole company, or even the other people dancing Giselle, to have watched those rehearsals, say, from the front of the house, and seen Karsavina demonstrate?"[88]

Shearer told Dale Harris that in 1948, at her first performance of *Giselle*, Cyril Beaumont, then critic for the *Sunday Times*, wrote "that a dancer of my appearance and coloring was really not acceptable in a role of this kind. As far as I can remember, he barely referred to either my dancing or interpretation. I remember feeling very depressed and rather angry."[89] Still, she had her fans. Arnold Haskell, for one, writing in 1949, excused her youth and the unfortunate lack of a really skilled partner (as Britain had suffered the loss of an entire generation of male dancers called up for wartime service). Haskell recognized her promise and suggested that Shearer's performance would only be heightened in the future. In his *Ballet Annual* for 1949, Haskell wrote of Shearer's July 13 performance that the ballerina had "fully proved her right to the honour of appearing as Giselle. She established the character from the very start and her early scenes were delightful." He quibbled with her mad scene, though, for it "requires a gentle mood at first as the simple character fails to understand what has happened to her and is groping in the darkness of lost memory." For Haskell, dramatic intensity in the mad scene should build gradually without ever becoming "a pathological study." The best ballerinas served "a long apprenticeship" in the work. He cited as evidence the superb performances of more mature ballerinas, including Yvette Chauviré, Fonteyn, and Alicia Markova. But Shearer was on her way to a fine interpretation, he said, for she was "blessed with the great gift of lightness that in the public's eye always excuses any technical shortcomings. This lightness is an enormous asset in the second act. She was not helped much by her partner either technically or dramatically, a fact that should be borne in mind."[90]

Another personal milestone for Shearer was the opportunity to dance George Balanchine's *Ballet Imperial*, which he set on the Sadler's Wells Company in 1950. Something of Shearer's style and personality made her respond with excitement to Balanchine's approach, and she recalled with pleasure her sole occasion to work with the choreographer. Unlike Fonteyn, Shearer had the light, deft fleetness that made her movement style more like that of George Balanchine's own American dancers. Shearer used her "slight and agile body well," noted Walter Terry, in the *Herald Tribune* for September 16, 1950. "Her movements are fluid, her phrasing better than that of many dancers and her leaps are deer-like in their lift and easiness." Mary Clarke explained the distinction between Fonteyn and Shearer, writing that Margot Fonteyn was "not naturally suited to the style" of Balanchine's choreography. Fonteyn was "above all a dancer who excels in choreography which has a heart," while, "Moira Shearer, on the other hand, had the right flash and brilliance and also the speed" required to dance *Ballet Imperial*.[91] James Monahan, another unabashed admirer of Fonteyn, explained Shearer's superior performance as a failure of *Ballet Imperial* itself, which he described as "unsatisfactory" and "arid." The ballet, he wrote, "requires of its ballerina a rare capacity for extremely rapid, intricate, terre-à-terre movement—for speed, in short. It is not that Margot Fonteyn has failed to cope even with this unsatisfactorily exacting role, but what used to be noticeable in the days when she and Moira Shearer alternated in it was that, in this one instance, the lesser dancer (possessed, however, of stronger feet and, consequently, of the greater gift for speed) did rather better than her more talented senior."[92]

There was clearly a mutual admiration between dancer and choreographer, and Shearer recalled her one experience with Balanchine as a highlight of her career.[93] She told Dale Harris that *Ballet Imperial* was exhilarating to dance and that she felt Balanchine treated her with respect and appreciation. Though she had been second cast in the role, she recalled, Balanchine made the unprecedented gesture of asking de Valois to provide him with a special rehearsal with Shearer. The rule, established by de Valois, was that only Fonteyn was allowed to work with outside coaches and choreographers. Shearer said it was "so pointless, so silly, and such a very great sadness to any of us who were second, third, or fourth because we were missing so much and we just had to try and pick up the pickings, you know. It was like being an Arab woman and eating the scraps that the men had left afterwards, and then the rest thrown to the dogs, and so on."[94]

With grave disapproval, de Valois granted Balanchine's request for a special rehearsal with the second cast. As Shearer recalled it:

Well, anyway, to go back to dear Mr. B. I arrived terribly early, good practice clothes, clean, tidy. And we started. I had listened to him very much in the early rehearsals, and I knew that he wanted this strange—the only way I can put it is—"offness" to everything. Instead of being straight up and down on your leg, he wanted you to give the impression that you were falling all the time; that it was all, instead of being upright. . . . You were at a diagonal. It was quite dangerous because if you didn't quickly get on to the other leg, and so on, you could literally fall. But you had to be at these angles—these dangerous angles all the time. Of course, it made it so exciting if you could do it. This was what I was so worried about; I didn't think I *could* do it.[95]

The ballet had a "tremendous added excitement of being dangerous," Shearer said, which came about because she was continually challenged to displace her center of gravity, a technical requirement that ran counter to all familiar classical ballet training. "And, my goodness," she added, "I had to sweat blood to be able to do some of those movements. But I've always found that fascinating to try. This is why I loved working with Balanchine so much. . . . He wanted something odd, and strange, and 'off,' classically 'off,' if you know what I mean, in quotes."[96]

Balanchine's gentlemanly demeanor and gentle urging worked magic, Shearer remembered:

> But what was so marvelous was that I remember absolutely—if I may put it like this—busting a gut for him at that first rehearsal. He said an absolutely sweet thing to me, which was enormously heartening. Then I could see his pleasure when he saw that I was getting this thing, and then he worked and he worked and he worked with me. He went on far longer than the time allotted to us. Then he said, "Are you tired? Are you tired?" I said, "No, no, not a bit," although I was absolutely dropping. But I thought, "What an opportunity. Here I've got this man all to myself, how wonderful." And the pleasure of doing it.

She acknowledged that although she had never felt secure with purely "technical" ballets, "to my amazement, because I so loved trying to do this funny odd thing that he wanted, and felt I was mastering it, I got such pleasure from it, and I adored dancing *Ballet Imperial* although it was so fiendishly difficult. But I loved it."[97]

HEIGHTENED WITH MEMORY

Moira Shearer passed away in 2006. Was it her fate to be remembered as the girl with the red hair who starred in that movie about the dancer? Shearer told Dale Harris that she often felt *The Red Shoes* preserved in celluloid an image of herself as an immature and not completely polished dancer. She described her sense that the film had dogged her:

> Well, as you know, that old movie roared around the world and then stayed in various places for years, and years, and years, and years. It was very difficult to be disassociated from it. I was terribly unhappy about my part in it because it was made—the dancing part of it particularly—just at a time when I was about to make a big stride forward technically and artistically, but I hadn't got there by any manner of means when this film was made. So, as a result, up there on the screen, which people still look at—and it still turns an old knife inside me to see it—is a particular kind of immature dancing which a year later had gone, I think, completely, and one was a totally different kind of dancer, and so much better in every way. However, there it was—I mean, that's life (laughs) That's the way it goes.[98]

Speaking with Harris in 1976, Shearer admitted to feeling a sense of regret. She believed she had never quite achieved that true sense of ease in classical technique. Looking back at photos and films of herself, she saw only "the spikey hands" for which she was often criticized. But there was one memory she shared with Harris that apparently struck a profound chord for her. She met a woman in a shop in Edinburgh, she said, who had remembered seeing her dance in *Cinderella*:

> She just gave me the feeling in what she said that maybe—and not necessarily for any of the right balletic reasons—but maybe one helped to create something that night for somebody which 25, 30, years later they still remember in a particular way. That, I think, is the reward for all the hard grindings and sloggings that one went through. It's marvelous if you feel, even if it was only for a comparatively small number of people, nevertheless it happened, and they've remembered something all their lives. Of course it's heightened with memory, and so on, which is very nice for the performer because you always seem better in people's memories than you actually were. This is the fatal thing about a movie. There it is in cold black and white, or color, and you can't get away from what was actually done.[99]

5
CATHERINE
KERR

I HAVE KNOWN Catherine Kerr since I arrived as a student at the Merce Cunningham Studio in New York City in the fall of 1981. At that time Kerr seemed remote and self-contained. Though we shared the same hallway and the same studios, and rode the same elevator, her workaday existence was off-limits for me. She was a serious—even severe, I thought at the time—member of the Merce Cunningham Dance Company. I could see her intensity every morning in class, and I felt that her work with Cunningham often drained her reserves of emotional and physical energy. Cunningham himself once wrote about the heavy demands of dance. "You have to love dancing to stick to it. It gives you nothing back, no manuscripts to store away, no paintings to show on walls and maybe hang in museums, no poems to be printed and sold, nothing but that single fleeting moment when you feel alive. It is not for unsteady souls."[1]

Watching Kerr rinse out her dance clothes in the sink in the late afternoons, and sensing her fatigue, I became curious about what she did in rehearsals, how Cunningham communicated with her, what challenges she confronted. I stood apart from the company's rehearsal regimen and wondered how that daily expense of physical activity resulted in dances that would spin excitement, energy, unpredictability, and beauty. The hairs on my arms bristled when I watched Cunningham's works on stage; but what was the intervening step?

How was it that those unbelievable dances emerged from the activities of a group of tattered, perspiring dancers who filed in and out of the large studio and who, after 5 P.M., showered, washed their leotards, combed their hair, smoked cigarettes, and went out to eat?

As I hung around the studio as a scholarship student, I wondered more and more how it happened that this group of people could become the Merce Cunningham Dance Company on stage. Did they feel the transformation when it happened? Did the dancing feel every bit as beautiful and spine-tingling as it looked? Something about Kerr's containment, her rigor, and her seriousness made me think she deeply felt the importance of what she was doing. To say I was in awe of Kerr would be to understate the silent respect I felt when I ended up alone with her—in the quiet of the small studio on a Saturday morning, or towel-clad, waiting for the shower. Then I joined the company and found that no one would talk about transformation. In the Cunningham ethos, there was no mystery, no stars, no rank, and no special status. Or, so goes the story.

These myths evaporated in the company dressing room. In the back room, by the windows, seated on the benches, behind the company bulletin board and next to the communal refrigerator, Kerr held a tacit rank. Her status had to do with her seniority, her longevity, and her sense of history. Kerr had stuck it out with Cunningham, and in spite of her youthful vulnerabilities, she had matured and endured, remaining committed for many years, more years, in fact, than most people managed to sustain the rigors of dancing for Cunningham. Kerr had some sort of unique, protean relationship with Cunningham that was difficult to define. He was the teacher, she the student; he was the courtly gentleman and she was his lady; he was the hunter and she was his prey. These attitudes shifted and overlapped, but they were all evident, at some point, in the choreography Cunningham devised for her.

Kerr grew up in the company; she was there during hard times as well as productive ones, and she had learned deeper and more substantial lessons from her tenacity. There was nothing unconscious or unreflective about Kerr, for as time went by, she developed a profound awareness of her place—which was significant—in the work. She did know a great deal about that work, and it was that I wanted to know from her.

Catherine Kerr was born on October 11, 1948, an "army child," she says, "which meant we moved every three or four years with each of my father's postings." One of five children, she started dance classes "because my mother said that was what you did with little girls." Ballet classes were a "running thread"

throughout family relocations from Georgia to Illinois to California, Germany, and Virginia. As a teenager, she trained for two years at the Washington School of the Ballet and one year at the National Ballet School in Washington, D.C., where dance and academic classes were included as part of an overall high-school curriculum. But her scholarship to the National Ballet School wasn't renewed because "I developed, as teenagers do." In retrospect she told me, "Perhaps if I'd been a better ballet dancer, the school might have kept me on through graduation." The whole hurtful experience surrounding her body image still troubled her years later. She gave a rueful laugh, and added, "It was the sixties, so you have to put it in context that, aside from the expectation that ballet dancers always be thin, this was also the era of Twiggy. Despite having great feet and long limbs, there did not seem to be a place for a curvy and athletically muscled body. When I developed, as teenagers tend to, there was a panic amongst the school teachers and my family at the change in my appearance." On the other hand, it may be that staying at the National Ballet School would not have been the right choice anyway. Kerr felt torn between the urge to dance and her desire to be a teenager, to spend time with her friends and to date. And there was confusion for her, too, in that she confronted "family expectations of college" and did not know how to satisfy these goals while pursuing a single-minded dance career. Ultimately, being a teenager won out and she switched to a public high school.[2]

Kerr's story evokes a sense of mainstream, middle-class America in which ballet classes were among the activities that parents afforded their daughters. Ballet might be included in an American middle-class girl's education as a way for her to learn gracefulness and to enhance her training in the arts, but there was to be no discussion of dancing professionally. There was something just too unreliable, too financially risky, and, for many families—with their legacies of American morality—too seedy and disreputable about a career on the stage. The assumption was that all the Kerr children would go to college, so her transfer to a public high school, and her subsequent education at the Pratt Institute in New York, were fully in line with her family's expectations.

At Pratt the dancing resurfaced, though this time it was classes in modern dance that engaged Kerr's intellect and fed her hunger for movement. She launched herself into modern dance workshops led by Pauline Tish, classes that attracted art and architecture students as well as dancers. "They were very lively, creative classes," Kerr recalled. "For someone who'd only had ballet, these workshops were both fun and a revelation." She had still further revelations when she began attending the experimental dance concerts that cropped up at various sites around Manhattan during the 1960s and 1970s. While a student at Pratt, Kerr saw dance concerts by Rudy Perez, Twyla Tharp, Yvonne Rainer, and the Grand Union. She first encountered Merce Cunningham's choreography in 1967 when she saw the Cunningham Company perform at the Brooklyn Academy of Music. "I remember seeing *How to Pass, Kick, Fall and Run* [1965], the Bruce Naumann piece with the fans, *Tread* [1970], and *Crises* [1961]. . . . I do remember the spirit of it," she said. "I saw *Rainforest* [1968]. I saw *Winterbranch* [1964]. I mean, it was an extraordinary introduction." As Kerr recognized, "It seemed more a reflection of the world than what I had seen in ballet. There was a seriousness of intent despite fans blowing, pillows floating around or people reading stories. The intensity . . . it was just extraordinary." Beyond the startling choreography, Kerr was drawn to the Cunningham dancers themselves, whom she called "awe-inspiring." Their dancing was "incredibly articulate," "elegant," "evocative and eccentric." Kerr said, "Those dancers ignited possibilities I didn't know existed in dancing." Her sense of awe stimulated new ideas about the possibilities of dance. But it also made her feel inadequate; at the time, she said, Cunningham's dancers seemed to represent a level of sophisticated virtuosity that she would never be able to achieve, and the choreography itself seemed highly "rarefied."[3]

On leaving Pratt with a liberal arts degree, she took a full-time job in a publishing company, but she harbored the notion that "it would be nice to choreograph, but not having any idea of what that meant." Eventually Kerr wound her way back into dance classes and was finally convinced by a friend to "Come to Merce's!" Kerr said, "A couple years after I'd finished college I had organized myself: I had a job, an apartment, and I had shed twenty pounds! Finally, I went and took Merce's, the six o'clock [elementary level] class. Merce was scheduled to teach. During the class, he gave me a correction. He stood right in front of me and did something with his chin. I didn't understand what he was doing, but I imitated him."[4]

Her anecdote spoke volumes about the relationship that would develop between the two over their years together: Cunningham demonstrating, Kerr imitating; Cunningham making a discrete but elusive correction, Kerr deciding how to respond and, in the process, giving life and movement to his suggestions.

Soon after she began taking classes at the Cunningham studio, the minimalist postmodern choreographer Laura Dean came to watch the class as she was looking for a group of dancers for her forthcoming tour to Europe. Kerr recalled, "She asked me if I would be interested in working with her. Well, I didn't know who she was from a hole in the wall. I said, 'Oh, yeah, sure.'" The adventure of working with Laura Dean and Dancers and Steve Reich and

Musicians would take Kerr away from the Cunningham studio for a year and a half. Touring with Dean and Reich was "great fun," Kerr remembered. "We had six shows in eleven weeks, so there was lots of time off." After working long hours at her editing job, assiduously attending dance classes at the close of work days, and somehow trying to sustain herself in New York City in the early 1970s, she said, "suddenly I was paid to be in Europe. I could go to museums and see pictures and have wonderful European food, and be an 'artist.'" Dancing with Dean, she explained, seemed "wildly eccentric." She continued, "You have to understand, I was of American midwestern, suburban background, and here I was in Europe, twirling like a dervish and stomping in circles, and getting paid!" Wryly, Kerr recalled that touring with Dean had seemed a wonderful life, but she was to realize, in later years, when she was "on a five-week tour with Cunningham, dancing six days a week and changing theatres every couple days," that being on the road with the Cunningham company was different. The Cunningham tours, she said, frequently left her "completely flat from fatigue, and required another level of commitment."[5]

When she returned to New York after her stint with Laura Dean, Kerr confronted the problem of trying to support herself given Dean's infrequent performance schedule. Living off the unemployment checks from her publishing job, she decided to return to the Cunningham studio and began to dabble in choreographing and producing concerts with a fellow dancer named Beth Blaskey. She was between jobs, figuring things out, taking dance classes and waiting for the next step in her life. So too, it turned out, was Cunningham. Kerr said, "In 1972 or 73, several dancers left Merce's company when Merce closed down the company. He had needed a break. During this lull, I stayed at Merce's, and was given a scholarship." Organizing her life around her job and her requisite scholarship classes was a struggle. "I took the advanced class, and another class in the afternoon. For approximately a year I did this crazy juggle. Oh, it was insane—if I hadn't gotten into the company, I don't know how much longer I could have kept it up."[6]

For Kerr this period marked a transition between her life as a student at the Cunningham studio and her subsequent invitation to join the company. But for Cunningham it was a hiatus of another nature as the choreographer was experiencing a shift in his relationship to his work and his company. In October 1972, Carolyn Brown, a longtime Cunningham dancer, gave her final performance with the company at the Théâtre de la Ville in Paris, ending her extraordinarily rich twenty-year partnership with Cunningham. "It was the end of an era," says David Vaughan, who notes that for two years after Brown's departure, the company performed only lecture-demonstrations, or "Events," as Cunningham called the hour-and-a-half-long performances designed for unconventional theater spaces. The small-scale, pared-down structure of these performances gave Cunningham some breathing room, so that he "did not have to address right away the question of a full repertory program without Carolyn Brown." For Cunningham, Brown's departure made "a profound change."[7]

During that period, too, Cunningham received an important commission from the Paris Opéra. In 1973 he spent nine weeks in Paris choreographing and also training the French ballet dancers in what became the "epic" *Un jour ou deux*. Cast for twenty-six dancers, the piece lasted more than ninety minutes without an intermission. It was first performed November 6, 1973, at the Salle Garnier in Paris. The large cast included the dancers Claude Ariel, Michaël Denard, Jean Guizerix, and Wilfride Piollet, all of whom had traveled to New York to study at the Cunningham studio before rehearsals began.

In another respite from the demands of creating repertory works for his company, Cunningham began at this time to explore his newfound interest in choreographing for the camera. Along with his collaborator Charles Atlas, Cunningham began to prepare a program of Events for CBS television's *Camera Three*.[8] This experiment would lead him to choreograph a number of works for camera through the decades of the 1970s, 80s, and 90s.

Each of these significant milestones in Cunningham's life—the departure of his friend, muse, and most important partner, Carolyn Brown; the opportunity to choreograph a substantial work on a world-class company of ballet dancers; and the choice to investigate the possibilities of dance on film and video—shaped the climate of the Cunningham Dance Company in which Kerr would work. The decades of the 1970s and 1980s would be radically distinct, too, from the preceding decades in that Cunningham would increasingly take himself out of performing. As he lightened his own performing load, he proportionally increased his concentration on choreographing for the ensemble, a change that drastically affected the look of the work.

In 1974 Kerr was asked into the company, and she remained to dance with Cunningham for three years. During her first period with the company she appeared in the 1974 work for video entitled *Westbeth;* she also danced in *Exercise Piece* (1975, created for Events) as well as in *Rebus* and *Sounddance*. She danced in the 1976 works entitled *Torse* (Part I) and *Squaregame,* and she left the company at the end of 1976 to marry a man who lived in Los Angeles. When that marriage never took place, Kerr decided to return to New York City. On Carolyn Brown's suggestion, she wrote to Cunningham and reentered the company. She then danced for Cunningham until her retirement from the company in May 1988.

When Kerr entered Pratt Institute as a student in the late 1960s, she had effectively launched herself into the center of a turbulent art world. Manhattan, and particularly Greenwich Village—the location of the Cunningham studio—was the nexus of sometimes brash and outrageous experimentation. For Kerr, coming from a middle-class American childhood, the artistic ferment of New York seemed outlandish, foreign, and intriguing. "The Village," particularly, bristled with a "revolutionary" energy as artists actively sought to undermine the status quo. Sally Banes explains that these artists, spurred on by antiwar activism, the civil rights movement, and the drug and sexual revolutions, were strongly attracted to novel ideas about who should make art and what constituted the making of art. The generation coming of age in the 1960s sought a "revolution," challenging what was valued as art, how art was conceived and produced, and what its effects should be. For many young artists, the goal was to use their art to alter the social fabric and change the culture in which they lived.[9]

By the 1970s when Kerr arrived at the studio, Cunningham was (in some circles) a sought-after teacher and much-admired choreographer. He had gained his status through his persistent, radical challenges to older, more established, or more traditional notions of dance composition. He and John Cage, his brilliant, frequently eccentric partner, collaborator, musical advisor, and mentor, met for the first time in the 1930s while Cunningham was studying at the Cornish Institute and Cage was on the faculty.[10] The two met again in New York City in the 1940s when Cunningham was dancing in the Martha Graham Dance Company. Under Graham's tutelage, Cunningham was schooled in a dramatic and emotive dance style.[11] After several years of training with Graham and performing her works, Cunningham grew disenchanted with the imposition of meaning and narrative on movement. Following Cage's lead in music composition, Cunningham came to believe that dance based on theme and variation and rooted in emotional or psychological meaning reflected an outdated view of art. Instead, he was intrigued by the movement possibilities inherent in the human body.

In the 1960s and 1970s numbers of musicians, visual artists, and choreographers were drawn to study composition with John Cage. And many dancers, who would eschew virtuosity and obvious dance technique in their own works, flocked to Cunningham's studio to study his technique.[12] Cage and Cunningham were inspired by the French Dadaist artist Marcel Duchamp (1887–1968), thought by some to be the greatest anarchist of them all. The creations of Duchamp—including the famous ready-mades—while often tongue-in-cheek or blatantly mundane, did provoke profound debates about the nature of art and its relationship to culture.[13] Like the older French artist, Cage embarked upon a lifetime of experimentation in which he would effectively upend fundamental notions of Western art. What Cage proposed, wrote Calvin Tomkins in 1965, was "the complete, revolutionary overthrow of the most basic assumptions of Western art since the Renaissance."[14] Influenced by lectures on Zen Buddhism offered by Dr. D. T. Suzuki, Cage began to reconsider the role of art in life. Abandoning many of the assumptions operative in Western culture concerning the making and reception of art, Cage and Cunningham, and others in their artistic circle, made works that resembled life processes in their seeming randomness, openness, and nonlinearity.[15] Such efforts to undermine all notions of "artistic and individual self-expression" found resonance among members of this younger generation of artists, who were also drawn to studying the philosophies and culture of the East.[16]

Cage's work challenged listeners to tune in to an environment of sound. Listening freely was prioritized over the creation of meaning or the packaging of experience in recognizable musical forms. In both his music making and his Zen Buddhist–inspired writings, Cage questioned "the power of art to communicate ideas and emotions, to organize life into meaningful patterns, and to realize universal truths through the self-expressed individuality of the artist." He avoided the artist's expression of individual creativity, proposing instead "an art born of chance and indeterminacy, in which every effort is made to extinguish the artist's own personality." Art—inseparable from life itself—was, for Cage, centered on "a perpetual process of artistic discovery."[17]

Similarly, Cunningham challenged time-honored assumptions about the orthodoxies of dance performance. Among other things, he explored novel ways to utilize stage space, and one of his most significant innovations, according to Sally Banes, was to dismantle inherited assumptions about theatrical perspective. He decentralized the dance space, stripping center stage of its heretofore unquestioned power. Cunningham perpetrated a "frontal attack on the picture-frame perspective that had been traditional, if not de rigueur, in dance performance at least since the eighteenth century." Doing away with the hierarchy of stage space, Cunningham created situations in which the spectator's eye could range freely from one dance activity to another. Instead of a picture frame, Cunningham created "an action field for dance" that resulted in a simultaneity of events, all of them of equal importance. This meant that observers could choose to watch one dancer over another as no one role was overtly privileged.[18]

Another orthodoxy exploded by Cunningham and Cage was that which united music and dance. Instead of conceiving of music and dance as necessary partners, Cage and Cunningham agreed to separate the two entities, determining only the time length of their otherwise autonomous compositions. Although the dance and music began and ended at the same time, the two elements were not necessarily aligned. Such a structuring principle allowed both elements to be developed fully, and it negated the imposition of "meaning" on the resulting compositions. The novel approach to collaboration gave Cunningham "a clear sense of both clarity and interdependence between the dance and the music."[19]

The same "blind" collaboration shaped Cunningham's relationship to the artists who designed his sets and stage pieces. Minimal guidelines were issued to all artists involved in any particular work. Each went off independently to create the music, the set, and the dance, and the elements came together only during final rehearsals. Surprisingly, Tomkins said, this approach did not "engender catastrophes." Instead, the melding of the elements created not a unified spectacle, but a collage, "in which disparate elements are brought together without becoming fused. We, the spectators, are invited to pay attention on three levels simultaneously, to hold in mind three separate forms and all the subtle reverberations among them." Attending a Cunningham performance was "as complex, as demanding, and as full of surprises as anything in our experience."[20]

Cunningham's approach to choreography was also shaped by his decision in the 1950s to experiment with the use of chance operations as compositional tools. Such activities as tossing coins, throwing the I Ching, or creating space charts allowed Cunningham to go beyond his own habits of unreflective composition: chance operations created a loose structure in which he, like Cage, could engage in what Cunningham called "a perpetual process of artistic discovery."[21]

Roger Copeland has described the importance, in Cunningham's ethos, of observing movement, and of the spectator's freedom to see in his or her own way. "Visibility in fact, was almost unlimited. It was a world that emphasized *seeing clearly* rather than *feeling deeply*."[22] While Cage's music led listeners to hear in new ways, Cunningham's dances prompted audiences to see differently. Rather than being asked to see dance as a narrative or dramatic vehicle, viewers entered into complex, often demanding and energetic spectacles that prioritized the visibility of bodies—most often clad simply and revealingly in unitards or leotards—moving in an open space.

What spectators also saw, and what Kerr noted in first attending performances by the Cunningham Company, was the "awe-inspiring" intensity and physical virtuosity of those Cunningham bodies. Early in his career as a choreographer, Cunningham found he had to prepare dancers to do the rigorous but elegant movement he was asking of them. Almost in spite of himself, Cunningham became a teacher, and, over the years, his classes yielded an identifiable technique. One of the few modern dancers of his generation to train in ballet, Cunningham studied ballet and taught modern classes for a time at George Balanchine's School of American Ballet. He was attracted to the ballet dancer's articulation of the legs and feet and discovered that ballet classes tended to cultivate strong legs and often enhanced dancers' ability to jump. In his own work, Cunningham drew from the ballet dancer's arsenal all that appealed to his interest in speed, spatial clarity, an articulated body, and complete physical mobility. In addition to the legs and feet of a ballet dancer, Cunningham valued a flexible spine, an active torso, and an emphasis on the body's ability to make quick changes of direction.

The characteristics of Cunningham technique were familiar to anyone who frequented dance concerts of the 1970s through the 1980s. Cunningham dancers were known for their swift weight transitions and their unexpected and lightning-sharp changes of direction. Viewer saw stillness broken up by flurries of activity. The dancers moved with a balletic elegance broken up by spurts of quirky, full-tilt awkwardness. The spectator's eye retained a sense that these Cunningham bodies were primarily vertical though they frequently indulged in twists, curves, and tilts off the vertical axis. Their fluid motion was often infused with raw energy as dancers abandoned refinement and charged through phrases of rhythmically complex arm and footwork. When there was unison ensemble work, the rhythms were often blatantly insistent, and shapes were clearly etched in space. There might be a lot of movement happening at the same time, making the viewer's task more complicated. As the stage space was opened up, the individual's focus was free to roam without conventional landmarks. Meanwhile, the dancers appeared unperturbed by all the activity as they executed highly complicated movement while maintaining, for the most part, detached, cool (some said mask-like) facial expressions.

In 1979, Una Flett, writing for the *Scotsman*, reported on an open class she witnessed at the Edinburgh Festival, commenting that one could see how "the body was being trained as a series of linked but independent components." Flett observed the way class exercises shaped dancers to Cunningham's style, which she described as "a peculiarly elegant hybrid of classicism and free eclectic movement." His youthful dancers were "endowed with the long beautiful line and high arched feet of ballet dancers. In addition, however, they have spines that can curl and stretch and twist like animals." The class was a "strange fantasy on a standard ballet class. Set above the strictest of correct placing in the basic foot and leg positions, all manner of bends and tilts are superimposed—all without benefit of a barre to hang onto."[23]

Cunningham once observed, "If the dancer dances—which is not the same as having theories about dancing or wishing to dance or trying to dance or remembering in his body someone else's dance—but if the dancer *dances,* everything is there. The meaning is there if that's what you want."[24] Catherine Kerr was a dancer who *danced.* She brought to Cunningham a ballet-trained body with a powerful physicality, an uncompromising readiness to take risks, and an unwillingness to hold back from dancing fully at every moment. A tall and strikingly handsome dark-haired woman, she had a long neck with a small head, deep-set eyes, and distinct facial features. Kerr's highly arched feet appeared to have a life of their own; she was loose-limbed with long legs and a flexible spine. She brought intelligence and a high degree of perfectionism to her work. Cunningham could rely on her to throw herself into any movement he cared to try out on her. He knew she would work fiercely to overcome obstacles. While other dancers might be daunted by the challenges he set, Kerr would dutifully set out to accomplish the task at hand.

From the beginning of her association with Cunningham, Kerr responded to the workmanlike pragmatism of the studio and the company. Technique classes were rigorous, drawing heavily on her early ballet training, and they were intellectually engaging. "She wasn't just a random dancer who had great legs," said Lise Friedman, a stunning dancer with a richly sensual movement quality who shared many years with Kerr in the Cunningham company.[25] "She really was mature—and educated. More educated than most dancers. And curious—very curious—and she fell in love, with the whole package." She was not simply a dancer anxious for a job. Friedman said Kerr's was "a much larger commitment" to the Cunningham aesthetic.[26]

The daily discipline of that training and the seriousness Kerr encountered at the Cunningham studio matched her own sense of responsibility to the work at hand. It was, after all, the way Cunningham approached his work. In an interview with Laura Kuhn, Cunningham invoked the commitment and discipline that for him and his dancers marked the center and focus of the profession. "In a dancer's life there's this constant discipline," he told Kuhn. "How you organize your life around the requirements of the dance thing, dance classes. Everything else you do has to be arranged to fit that structure."[27] Bound as she was by a sense of loyalty to Cunningham and of responsibility to the movement he gave her, Kerr would never rest easily with her own performances. She would push herself to exceed her own limits, displaying a rigor that matched Cunningham's own and that allowed him to further his fascination with the possibilities for movement inherent in her body and personality.

The new dancers entering the company in the 1970s came in with what Lise Friedman described as "a lot of ballet training" or, as in Kerr's case, they felt pushed by the challenges of the choreography to "go back" to ballet class. The new generation could "take the choreography farther than it had been taken before, technically," said Friedman. Cunningham was "tuned into the world around" him, and with his developing fascination with film and video, he was able to "explore the idea that movement was faster on film, and how the space changes, and I think all of that fed into his appetite for speed." It interested him to utilize fully the dancer/tools at hand: "if you can run across the room faster than another person, then he's going to have you run as fast as you can. If he wants to see a leg that goes this high—maybe he can see it go even higher. If you can do a deep back bend, maybe you can go even farther." In rehearsals he continued to prod and push to see what more could be achieved by his extraordinarily skilled and able dancers: "'Can you try that?' 'Can you do that?' 'What would happen if you did that?' Always pushing, always interested to see one more—you know, pushing the envelope is what makes him a great choreographer. The world was moving faster."[28]

The world was moving faster and the technique classes were becoming even more demanding—there were more balances, more turns, higher legs, more quick beaten jumps—as Cunningham became known for training and hiring virtuoso dancers. But, while it was clear his dancers had technique, some viewers thought that was all they had. By the 1970s and 1980s, during Kerr's years with the company, Cunningham's status as an important experimental choreographer was no longer in question; however, some critics complained vociferously that his work had become cerebral or mechanical. They alleged that the younger generation lacked the quirky eccentricity, warmth, and humanness noticeable in the dancers of the 1960s. In an essay written in the late 1970s, David Vaughan acknowledged what many observers had already noted: there was a shift in emphasis in Cunningham's choreography. Beginning in the 1970s—corresponding with Carolyn Brown's departure from the company and the choreographer's experience working with the large group of French ballet dancers cast in *Un jour ou deux*—Cunningham demonstrated a new concern with "mass effects." He reformulated the company, adding Kerr and other new dancers to make pieces "in which longer passages of unison choreography occur," and in which "individuals do not stand out even when everyone on stage is doing something different." Vaughan took issue with the criticisms that the younger dancers seemed to lack the "strong personalities" of the earlier generations; on the contrary, Vaughan said, the company of the 1970s perfectly matched Cunningham's "present concerns as a choreographer." What Cunningham demanded from the dancers of Kerr's generation was "virtuoso movement." The dancers brought to the creative process "pure technique," such as "swiftness of execution and the elimination of transitions between one movement or position and another." While it might seem contradictory, Vaughan said, Cunningham drew out the individuality of his dancers since "everyone in the world walks according to the same mechanism, but no two people walk alike, and that is what constitutes 'expression.'"[29]

Another shift in the choreography came with Cunningham's diminished presence on the stage. As Cunningham aged, his own difference from his dancers became increasingly evident in the work. Often Cunningham created his own roles so as to play off this distinction in ages. *Rebus*, created in 1975, was, according to Cunningham, "a dramatic dance lasting thirty-one minutes, with me as protagonist, in opposition to the young dancers of my company acting as chorus." Vaughan explained that *Rebus* was the first work to highlight "the generational difference between Cunningham and the rest of his company." In this dance, Cunningham appeared "as a detached, controlling presence, setting choreographic puzzles and equations for his dancers to solve."[30] As Cunningham aged, his dancers functioned more and more as a youthful "chorus." They were strong, technical dancers whose energy and physicality increasingly offset the dramatic figure of the choreographer moving with them, but always separated from them onstage.

Jim Reed, writing for the *Woodstock Times* in June 1980, spoke to both Cunningham's dramatic presence and the individual personalities of his dancers. "Cunningham's dancers have markedly distinct stage personalities and in all of the choreographed pieces are free to express them uncurbed. Their differences do not disturb the structure of the dance; they contribute to its definition. The only masks are the dancers' natural masks." In fact, Reed observed frequent onstage communication and exchanges between the dancers, who demonstrated awareness of their relatedness in space: "Easy personable exchanges between individual dancers (never uniform or pervasive) occur frequently and naturally. A few of the dancers move in an icy remoteness, seemingly indifferent to each other or to us. (Some of us want to be acknowledged strictly on our merits.)"[31]

Reed described the way Cunningham could be seen to wander among his youthful dancers, who were moving vigorously and at full tilt around him:

Cunningham amid his troupe, totally alone in his age, elfin in the delicacy of his every gesture, powerfully communicates an image of immortality that is at once poignant and joyous: the guru-teacher moving with ethereal grace among the vigorous physical triumphs of his dancers, who do now with exuberant ease what he once did and taught them to do. A compelling passage in *Squaregame* shows the choreographer standing enigmatically behind an impassioned solo by Cathy Kerr, his right hand raised over her exertions, his fingers moving subtly, like a master at his universal work.

Impassioned, daring, committed, Kerr began to emerge as a striking, if grave and intensely focused, presence on stage. Critics noted her passage from "unrelieved virtuosity" to her gradual assumption of control and self-assertion onstage. In 1974 Kitty Cunningham remarked on Kerr's obvious newness to the work and her "beautiful balletic technique."[32] By 1980 Alistair Macaulay found Kerr "austere" and commanding.[33] Edward Willinger, in his review of *Coast Zone* (1983–84) at City Center in New York, called her "outstanding" and noted her "stern, deadpan manner, heavy thighs, and high, powerful, grand battement."[34] The tenor of the reviews changed as critics began to account for her power and her womanliness. Janice Berman, writing in the March 28, 1983, issue of *Newsday*, described a particularly vivid moment in Event Number 2 at City Center, noting "Catharine [*sic*] Kerr's duet with Joseph Lennon, where she seems at once a madonna and a crucified figure." Deborah Jowitt, commenting on Kerr's development as a performer, wrote in the *Village Voice* for March 25, 1986, "Speaking about Cunningham's remarkable company is often as difficult as speaking about the blend of immediacy and enigma in his works. Granting all his dancers' great technical facility, clarity, and lack of mannerism, the highest praise I can ever find to give is that they look 'like themselves.'" Jowitt remarked on the "beautiful, sometimes drastic duet" for Alan Good and Catherine Kerr in the 1985 dance entitled *Arcade*. It was "drastic" because Good "throws her straight up and lets her slip quite low before he catches her." Jowitt observed, "What happened opening night was quite extraordinary. Kerr, who never seems to have the confidence you'd think her beauty, accomplishment, and experience would engender, gradually came alive during this duet. I saw it happen, or rather felt it happen, and I think I stopped breathing."

Though Kerr's rank was only tacitly acknowledged, over the years Cunningham did recognize her uniqueness for he often cast Kerr as his partner in large, full-company works. One of the dances that most beautifully featured Kerr with Cunningham as her partner was *Duets* (1980). Cunningham told Jacqueline Lesschaeve that *Duets* spun out of an initial dance for a man and a woman, created for Event performances. "Having finished that one, I decided to make a second, and then a third for other dancers in the company, until there were six."[35] The costumes were designed by Mark Lancaster, "who put the women in short skirts. Each dancer wore a color that was picked up in the costume of a dancer in one of the other couples."[36] The choice to costume the women in skirts highlighted the play on the structure of the familiar ballet *pas de deux*.

In her February 25, 1980, *New York Times* review of the premiere, Anna Kisselgoff described the new warmth she observed in the choreography: "A duet is traditionally a metaphor for a relationship between a man and a woman," she wrote. "If Mr. Cunningham's work normally leads us to regard his choreography as pure movement, the atavistic love connotation of the duet tradition nonetheless makes itself felt in *Duets*. The result is a special human warmth and glow uncommon in recent Cunningham pieces." Noting that each duet had "its own distinctive movement signature," she observed the novel partnering techniques explored in the Cunningham-Kerr "central" duet. The choreographer seemed to be "constantly adjusting the angles of her wrist, hand and so forth." For Kisselgoff, the duet suggested a master choreographer rethinking and editing his work. In this reading, Kerr's function was to serve as his responsive young dancer, always moving in accord with his directions, corrections and revisions.

Robert Greskovic also saw the duet as playing out a relationship between the artist and his materials: "In his own duet with Catherine Kerr, there's a moment when she stands in relevé passé with one arm raised straight up out of her tilted torso. After steadying Kerr in her pose, Cunningham then focuses on that vertical arm. He alternately grabs, pats, and tags her arm from shoulder to wrist. It could be seen as a hand-over-hand climb to claim a baseball bat, but I prefer, for my purposes here, to see it as a sculptor patting the finishing touches onto the clay of a sculptured arm."[37]

In October 2001, Kerr had just returned from setting the work on dancers at the Ballet de Lorraine. The experience of teaching *Duets* to a group of dancers unfamiliar with the Cunningham repertory objectified the dance somewhat and allowed Kerr to see her own duet in a new light. She said, "While teaching *Duets* just now, I saw within the duet he made for us that the duet was not only about the 'master choreographer' working with the younger dancer, but that the duet also dealt with my habit of falling, tripping, wobbling, or being 'down,' and his assisting me through these moments. I thought it was a humorous and tender comment on our own relationship. When he grabbed either of my arms at the end, while I was tilted in passé, he would lift me up." She recalled an instance in technique class when "Merce just came over to me and hauled me up on my leg to try to teach me how to lift up *on* my leg." She added, "I look back at that duet, and I realize that from the opening *plié* and the reach out, the duet is also about falling, and recovering from being down."[38]

Could it also have been about her daring? About her proclivity for launching herself into space and taking risks? I raised this point with Kerr, and she replied,

> Yes, I think so. In that duet there's a point where, while quickly rising and turning in place, the woman flings her leg, and an arm, up to the side three times. On the third fling, she tilts side and falls—down. The leg swings high, higher, highest, and then the torso tilts. The rhythm's accent changes from up to down. Merce never explained it to me as a fall. He said, "Take it [the leg] up, and up, now, down, down, *plié. Down, up, down, up, down.* He never used the word—so I never thought of it as falling—I never translated it, when I was thinking about it—as falling. When he taught the section where I did the leaps, he said, "Take your back forward," after I landed, which deepened the *plié.* I realized that it was about leaping and falling and the partner/teacher/Merce running to pull, assist, or lift me.

Whatever other human interactions and relationships might emerge for spectators, for Kerr the duet is about "two people together, one assisting, supporting the other."[39]

In *Doubles,* Kerr's role again seemed extraordinary; her power in the role Cunningham devised for her drew audience attention to her opening solo and seemed to give it dramatic weight.[40] The work opened with Kerr (or, in the alternate cast, Friedman) alone onstage. As the curtain opened, the dancer extended her leg into the space in a slow and weighty adagio. That so many observers saw Kerr's role as central had much to do with her physical commitment to the choreography, for what could have been a simple adagio sequence became a defining moment. A structural principle at work in *Doubles* was the superimposition of solos with duets and trios so that separate activities were often going on at the same time. Viewers saw simultaneous movement in the foreground and background areas of the stage. But there was another sort of doubling going on as well; the company was literally split into two casts, each maintaining its own considerably different version of the dance. The music was by Takehisa Kosugi (*Spacings*), and the costumes, consisting of leotards and close-fitting sweatpants, were designed by Mark Lancaster. Unlike Cunningham's large group works of that time, *Doubles,* cast for half the company, seemed a relatively quiet, small-scale piece. For Friedman, it was "almost a step back" in time for Cunningham. "I thought that he had cleared the stage off and he had gone back in time in a way. Not that it was old-fashioned, but he had gone back to an earlier idea about stage space."[41]

Kerr's striking opening solo drew nearly unanimous praise. Julie Kavanaugh, writing in the *Spectator*, observed that Kerr displayed "a wonderful pliant grace." Jennifer Dunning in the *New York Times* called the dance "one of Mr. Cunningham's happiest inventions." Dunning described that opening adagio: "The dance begins with the quietly lyrical Catherine Kerr alone on stage, serenely marking out 'Cunningham territory' with her long, stretched, curving limbs and pulled-up body. Two men sprint on, and the pull begins between that grave lyricism and the scuffed-jump roistering. It is a gentle pull." The "pull" that Dunning observed gave the choreography a rich texture. "It is fascinating to watch the difference in attack among the men alone. . . . A brief duet for Miss Kerr and Mr. Swinston is filled with those wonderful Cunningham stops, sudden, neat and punctuating."[42]

Tobi Tobias described the company's first New York performance of *Doubles*, at City Center in 1985. Tobias was enthralled; she was particularly enthusiastic about Kerr's solo, referring to the dancer as "long-limbed and full-hipped—a nature goddess," who opened the dance by "carving her way through the space." Next, "as if she had summoned them, two men run on, jump straight up and down, and fall to the ground, ears pressed to the earth for subterranean messages." Tobias described the later duet in which Kerr ran hand-in-hand across the space with Robert Swinston. "Swinston supports her in exquisite, tenuous adagio poses, but intermittently there's this frantic running, as if they were fugitives, or lovers rushing for a secret shelter."[43] For Alan Kriegsman, Kerr's movement had an animal-like quality. He described a "tall, willowy Catherine Kerr poised in waiting, alone on stage. She begins to move, slowly, her arms angling into mysterious signals, her torso folding forward, her leg rising in a breathtaking arc, and the movement takes on a quality of animal stealth."[44] Mindy Aloff, though more matter of fact about the work, saw the solo as "a fine vehicle for displaying Kerr's sumptuously arched feet and powerful thighs."[45]

In her Cunningham-like self-deprecation, Kerr refused—when pressed—to comment on the variety of images critics saw in her dancing. She preferred to focus on the work and the tasks Cunningham had set for her. Describing the choreographic structure of *Doubles*, she explained that "the whole solo was counted on one. Merce was specific during the rehearsal period that each movement take one count and be separate. That was the way it was taught. 'Circle your arm: one. Take a step: one.'" In her private rehearsals with Merce, she said,

> some instructions were verbal, "Could you try . . ." but, he actually got up from his chair at certain points—when he was working with me—and would do

a step. My response when I was around Merce was always to try to do what he was doing, to attempt to imitate his rhythm or shape. The rhythm of what he set up was every weight shift was a count, that is, from foot to foot, or bending or straightening, or rising on a leg. The movements weren't to go together, but were to be distinct. There would be points when there would be an extension to the side, which I found altered the tempo. The emphasis on separating each movement established an effect, or quality of deliberateness. That made it meditative—the deliberateness of it.[46]

Where then does the power come from? Kerr said, "I imagine it was a quality of the dance's movements on my body; how the instructions I was given were displayed by the quality of my muscles, ligaments and bones, my physicality. And the fact that you're on the stage! Merce never talked to me about 'quality.' However, if you know that your circling arm is the only gesture that's occurring on the stage at that time and you're sharing the space with Kosugi's music, I think you make it . . ."[47]

Perhaps the word she was searching for was "powerful."

Another major role for Kerr can be seen on a videotape recording of Cunningham's *Points in Space* (1986), shot in a television studio at the BBC. The documentary recording of the work plays on the possibility of multiple perceptions, using a slowly scanning camera that dislocates the viewer from any fixed point in space. Camera work and choreography interact to create an ongoing sense of movement. Groups or solo dancers move in and out of view of the camera, and the dance feels as if it continues just outside the range of vision: if you move slightly away from your fixed point, you will see another dance from another perspective.

The piece opens with three women in a triangular, or V, formation. One man is seen behind and to the right of the women; he is poised in a lunge on one knee, his back curved and one arm extended. Another man enters and, in a series of staccato jumps, moves between and around the women, who continue to turn and swing their legs in wide sweeps around their bodies. Suddenly, the women in the V formation whisk out of the camera's lens, revealing now three men who swing their legs in arcs, as they spring off the floor and circle their arms. The sections alternate fast and slow tempos. Kerr, dressed in a royal blue unitard, is seen primarily in slow, adagio sections in which she most often moves steadily from one perched *relevé* balance to another. Slowly, smoothly, she and her partner—they are offset by another duet couple moving through a different series of partnering actions—appear to exist in a heavy, dense interplanetary atmosphere. Kerr shapes the arcing of her leg around her partner so that she straddles his back.[48] Swinging her leg in a smooth *grand rond de jambe,* she circles it behind her partner, leans against him, and laces her arms behind her, through his extended arms. Holding her only by one hand, he slowly lowers her down to the floor as she tilts fully to one side. She descends to the floor, supporting herself on one knee with the other leg extended open and to the side, and props herself—still holding her torso in a tilt—on one hand. The camera lingers briefly over this shape and then continues its steady panoramic sweep to pick up other moving bodies in the space.

When the dance was performed as a stage work in 1987, several changes had been made. Cunningham's role was omitted and some sections were reorganized or cut. Alistair Macaulay noted the changes in Kerr's duet, now danced with Alan Good. Macaulay commented on the new sense of drama in the duet, calling it "now the work's high point":

> In one sequence, twice repeated, Kerr is held under her armpits by Good so that her seat is near the floor (it's like Leto's two handmaidens in the Prologue of Balanchine's Apollo, if you can remember that); then she sweeps one leg out and around, pins down that foot to the floor, and pulls herself and Good in that direction. The passage has a drama reminiscent not of Apollo but of some great duets from other Balanchine ballets. So does the backbend she does in his arms, in which she walks forward, unseeing, advancing one leg through high forward developpé before planting it and moving on. This being Cunningham, each duet keeps changing its drama. One feels the relationship forever new, although it has certain constants in Good's handsome presence, the tender strength of his partnering and Kerr's austere authority.[49]

Kerr undoubtedly had a large commitment to Cunningham and to the movement he gave her. Dancing with Cunningham was "work," and, Kerr said, it was only later that she started realizing she was "an artist." Work constituted the core of her experience. It meant, she said,

> that you get out there and try as hard as you can to do the movement you've been given to the best of your ability. Which means, and this is a gift I think from Merce to his dancers—it's a terrible, terrible burden too—but it's also his great gift, that where you are at that point in your life, where you are in your understanding is what you present to the world, what you bring to the material he hands you. Whether you're struggling with work that was made on another body, with a different history and sensibility than your own, or if you're creating something in the moment with him.[50]

The struggle to bring movement to its fullest realization reflected Cunningham's approach to his own work. "This is the example that Merce gives us," Kerr said, and "what's difficult for the dancers is that you have this phenomenal example from this man who obviously has profound gifts, really, that separate him from the rest of us. Because he sets up such an example for us by how he approaches his work that ... my feeling was that the expectation was that we return that. ... It was so intense. ... The atmosphere [of the studio] always felt so intense. I wish I could have laughed more."[51]

Friedman noted that Kerr may have been more sensitive to the level of intensity and commitment than were most dancers. She suggested Kerr unconsciously felt the pressures of being the woman whom Cunningham singled out most often to be his partner. "I think she was under a lot of pressure because Merce was kind of in love with her—infatuated with her—and it put pressure on her in a way that she couldn't shrug it off. I mean, to be sought out as his partner, to have this kind of intense relationship with him. That's a lot of pressure. It's a lot to bear."[52]

Kerr acknowledged that she had felt pressure. She struggled to understand the extraordinary relationship she had with Cunningham.

> Of course, I was extremely flattered. I mean, I was always aware that, of course, I wasn't Carolyn [Brown] or Viola [Farber], because I wasn't his peer. I always thought that every duet played on the master-student relationship, whether it was *Squaregame* [1976] or in *Rebus* [1974] or *Roadrunners* [1979]. Why me? Physical match in size? Merce is a very visual person and he looks at bodies in that way. Chemistry?—When Merce taught his part [in *Duets*] to Robert [Swinston], he actually said to Robert, "You're prowling," as he promenades the woman in attitude. Then Merce looked at me and smiled. Well, I had always sensed that. So there must have been some kind of *frisson* that I suspect was part of his creative imagination.[53]

Particularly notable among Kerr's other partnerships in the company was her pairing with Joseph Lennon. Friedman speculated on the unique chemistry between Kerr and Lennon. "I think Joseph humored her and Joseph calmed her down. And I think Joseph brought out a lot of 'coltish' qualities in her dancing." Friedman added, "She always had that 'starting-gate agitation' about her which I think interested Merce."[54]

Physically the two were well matched. Friedman said, "She could also be very grand on stage—you know she is big." Kerr's serious demeanor, dark hair, pale skin, and height made the handsome, dark-haired Lennon "more assertive in a way, because he had to be there. Not that Cathy couldn't balance on her own, but the duets were constructed in such a way that she really needed Joseph's support. I mean Merce would have her *fall* into Joseph's arms. Over and over again."[55]

And Lennon's more playful, relaxed attitude balanced Kerr's intense concentration. Friedman said,

> Well, I think Merce has a very devilish side, and he not only sees someone's strengths, he also sees someone's weaknesses. And I think Merce kind of toyed with her combativeness and her inability to compromise in rehearsal, much of which came out of her incredibly overblown commitment to his steps. With her, it was never, I want to do these steps this way, but I fully believe it to be this way, and I want to do it the way it should be done. And of course, that could be maddening for everybody, but also very wonderful and very endearing. She was often very much on edge in rehearsal.[56]

When the company first saw Kerr in rehearsal, paired with Joseph Lennon in the 1978 work entitled *Exercise Piece Duet,* she recalled that many remarked,

> "Oh how perfect." It was like a playful game of tag in the section where the woman steps out in arabesques darting across the stage and the man has to jump side to side to tap one arm and then the other arm. Initially I stepped out too far for Joseph to get around me. That wasn't usually the case for me with Joseph. Most often I felt I had to dash to keep up with him. Joseph's request that I not step out so far amused me, because Joseph always moved out, as big as he could. And the things Merce made Joseph do! Merce asked if it would be "possible" for me to dive into a curved over turn and then fling myself backward. "And Joseph will catch you." Merce then instructed Joseph to run around me while I turned, "And catch her." We all laughed, and then gave it a try. It was always terrifying and exciting to do for me as well as for the person who had to catch me. I just think Merce found it very exciting to have two dancers who always took things to the edge. That was not something that I consciously tried to do, it was just how I danced.[57]

Kerr danced with an alert, edgy power and an utter commitment to the task Cunningham set for her. But critics also noted her womanliness and, increasingly, those of us who watched her felt an emotional undertow in her dancing. Her changing relationships with Cunningham may have had something to do with the shifts in her various roles. Laura A. Jacobs called her a "lioness of a dancer."[58] What Maggie Lewis observed in a performance of *Phrases* (1984) was Kerr's "workmanlike" quality, and a complex, shifting relationship with Cunningham:

The workmanlike feeling came across strongly—almost humorously—when Cunningham himself appeared with Catherine Kerr in a pas de deux with all the wind taken out of its sails. He gave Kerr his hand to lean on, but instead of gazing absorbedly at her as she turned, stretched, and balanced, he faced the audience straight on and deadpan. In ballet, partnering hides the dancers' efforts so they only seem to be standing close to each other because they're so in love. Cunningham was obviously there to give Kerr a hand. . . . They were so sturdily cooperative, Kerr's poised strength almost went unnoticed. Almost. The plain effort and support were more touching than romance. Entering and leaving the stage, Cunningham and Kerr held hands. On the way in, Cunningham seemed to be leading a student. As they left, the powerful Kerr gave him her hand as if looking after her teacher.[59]

By the late 1980s, Kerr knew she would soon leave the company. "I had finally gotten to a point where I enjoyed being on stage and felt satisfaction with my dancing," she said. But she "recognized it was time to go," as she found herself working with dancers who were, for the most part, considerably younger than she. Ironically, this new sense of happiness allowed her both to "relax on stage" and to "blossom into other relationships in her life." She married Joshua Ginsberg, a wildlife ecologist, in 1988.[60]

She and her husband moved to England in 1988. From that home base, she frequently traveled to join him in Zimbabwe, where he ran a project on African wild dogs. The couple returned to New City in 1996.

Since leaving the company, Kerr returns to teach at the Cunningham studio upon occasion and has been on the faculties of the California Institute of the Arts, the London Contemporary Dance School, the Laban Institute, and the Conservatory of Dance at the State University of New York at Purchase. She has been asked to teach and stage some Cunningham dances for the Rotterdam Dansgroep, Charleroi/Dances, Ballet Opera de Paris, Rambert Dance Company, Maggio Danza, and the Ballet de Lorraine.

MEMORIES OF KERR

When I call up my own memories of Kerr in any number of her roles—the trio from *Torse* (1976), for instance, which was frequently performed in Events—I recall first an image of her articulate feet and legs. She has a flexible and fluid spine but holds herself high in the chest, lifted above the diaphragm. She shows incredible rigor about doing the movement with clarity and "as it should be," even at the expense of occasional awkwardness or tension in the body.

She doesn't smooth out the edges but moves with power as she is propelled through the air by her two male partners. In a solo such as that at the opening of *Doubles,* though, she is capable of an exquisite, meditative lyricism, showing beautiful, unforced leg extensions and calm steadiness and control. Her legs move high, and in her *grands ronds de jambes*—big sweeps of the leg in a circular pattern—they swing with a force that reminds me of the pendulum of a grandfather clock. She is grounded and weighted through her pelvis, but she is also capable of appearing suddenly deft, mobile, and fleet. She pushes through molecules in the atmosphere when she travels. There is weight and force to her legs, daring and power. Kerr is majestic, not light.

One of the most compelling aspects of watching her dance was the almost childlike way she drove herself to "get it right," the gravity of her attention to doing the movement as it was given to her. In Cunningham's solar system, the focus was on the work, and the company was presented to the public as the Merce Cunningham Dance Company, a collection of relatively anonymous "supertechnicians of dance" who were gathered to "see how the movement operates . . . how you get from this position to the next one, and move everything from there," as Cunningham put it.[61]

Nevertheless, in spite of the "democratic conceptions of art and artist," individual dancers have made their marks on key roles, leaving traces of their bodies and their distinct movement qualities in their roles and in the memories of observers, critics, and fellow dancers.[62] In reality, Kerr told me, it was the personhood of the individual dancer, fulfilling to her utmost the movement as given, that shone through and attracted the notice of onlookers. What shone through Kerr were her courage and vulnerability, her ability to take risks on stage and in life, and her utter conviction that dancing well was a critically important human endeavor. These are the qualities that linked her to Cunningham; they fill out his choreography and give humanity and physicality to the works he would not have created without her.

EPILOGUE

WHEN I WAS A YOUNG and hopeful dancer in New York during the 1970s and 1980s, an unchallenged certitude hovered over my daily experience: as a female dancer I knew I was entirely replaceable. If I tore a cartilage in my knee, compressed the disks in my spine, sprained an ankle, or broke a bone in my foot, there always another highly talented woman who could take my place. It drove me and all the women dancers I knew to ambitious efforts to excel. We all longed to "get work," receive juicy parts, be noticed by our teachers and choreographers. We hoped that by perfecting our technique, shaping and honing our bodies, and improving our mental capacities—by making ourselves seen among all the others—we would somehow be afforded the opportunity to dance. It has never been an easy way to live.

Although there have been changes in the cultural and social contexts in which female dancers have trained and performed throughout two hundred years of history in the Western world, this sense of one's redundancy and the drive to excel have not changed. For the most part, dancers' goals and desires remain much the same. Paradoxically, in spite of the immense efforts female dancers make and have made throughout history to stake out careers, they have a limited number of years available to work as performing artists. They mature early, peaking as dancers often before they have resolved the confusions of youth. Few of them will ever claim to have altered or shaped the development of dance.

But in spite of the brief span of their careers and the ephemeral nature of their contributions, dancers themselves are the elements from which dance history is made. Change happens incrementally in the daily regimen of a dancer's life, although history records only the final products of the experiments and innovations worked out through their bodies. Historical milestones are recorded as a result of an ongoing dynamic process in which female dancers respond to demands in their dance classes and rehearsal studios, govern their choices according to the most vibrant artistic debates, and eke out their existence according to the most compelling economic concerns of their times. In this equation, dancers both create possibilities and respond to the circumstances surrounding their careers. Despite the brevity of their professional lives, their practiced bodies create the look of the dance of the day and help to determine—as much as they respond to—the larger aesthetic debates that inform their art.

In the face of its evanescence, the dance of the past is, of course, vastly difficult to recuperate. On the other hand, while writing about dance can be problematic, and recording dance is fraught with hardships, such challenges are not insurmountable. In order to approach an understanding of the role of the dancer in creating and shaping the dance of the past, it is important to consider the dynamism and the complexity of the form; it is a performing art that comes to fruition within a particular set of economic, social, and cultural contexts. It is purveyed by specialized bodies trained through a system of practices that are themselves responsive to a culture's aesthetic, scientific, and artistic theories. In turn, dance is received by audiences of widely varying composition who interact with what they see both as individuals and as members of larger social communities. Records of dance's past can be extricated—admittedly with some difficulty—from these overlapping, intertwining systems. The past, Alexandra Carter writes, "exists only in records of the events, not in the events themselves." Thus, the "interrogative and imaginative task of the historian" is to give meaning to the records of the past. But, she asserts, dance history lacks an acknowledgement of the role of the dancers who create the events. A complex, dynamic history that accounts for the contributions of the dancers themselves still needs to be written. "We know about the big names," Carter writes, "and we will probably never know the actual small names, but we can be alert to the notion that the dance event is produced not only by individual creative artists but by unacknowledged armies of dancers, walk-ons, administrators, scene builders and movers, front-of-house, publicity and marketing people and so on. We cannot, as said, name all these but we can acknowledge that context is not just background, but context is what produces the artistic event, and shapes our perception of it."[1]

My purpose here is not to give names to the nameless, but instead to recreate the world of a handful of dancers and to recognize their contributions to the dance of their times. My goal has been to examine a portion of Western dance history by analyzing—as closely as possible—the workaday lives of five women dancers whose careers transpired during significant periods of Western dance. I have attempted to uncover their physical experiences and to take one step closer to an embodied history of dance.

Such an investigation involves the historian in making some imaginative leaps, as Carter predicted, for history at the body level is all but impossible to record. In cases prior to the availability of film and video products, I have turned to literary records—including poems and criticism—and to various forms of iconography, among them painting and sculpture. All of these resources must be treated with caution as they are themselves the creative products of artists rather than conscious efforts to accurately record dance. Most often these sources give us impressions, memories, and the spirit of the thing itself. However, while dealing judiciously with the riches of history and being sensitive to idealized representations, we can use these documents to get closer to an understanding of the dance of the past.

On the other hand, there are pitfalls in relying only on videos and films; while poetic and critical writing might communicate the spirit of the dance at the expense of the hard data, films and video often convey the data without the spirit. As Moira Shearer observed, "this is the fatal thing about a movie. There it is in cold black and white, or color, and you can't get away from what was actually done." A wider scope is often necessary to evaluate fully the dancer's impact, as a film records (as Shearer put it) the "spikey" hands while resisting the full dimensionality of her moving body. Given the difficulties attendant on the process, however, there is much to be gained by reenvisioning a history through the stories of individual dancers, for we recapture the sense that dance is made through a dynamic, interactive process, that it is an ongoing activity and is not completely represented by the performance landmarks customarily recorded in history.

There are several commonalties in these five women's careers spanning two hundred years, similarities that reinforce the essential elements of the profession. Each woman was deemed physically attractive according to the standards of beauty of her era, a quality that contributed substantially to her career as a performer. Each was physically gifted and worked with extraordinary discipline from an early age to command a large measure of control over her body. Sometimes, though, the women's bodies were recalcitrant or slowed the forward momentum of their career goals. Baccelli's several pregnancies interrupted her career at various times, though only one child, a son, lived beyond infancy. Karsavina acknowledged she suffered periods of overwork and frailty that necessitated dosing with special tonics and, at one time, a period of complete rest and convalescence. Shearer was "plagued" by her red hair and porcelain skin and was often told she was too "light" to perform the classics. Kerr felt self-doubt for a time when teachers and family told her she lacked the ideal ballet dancer's body.

Differences in cultural contexts also emerge, as the social role of the dancer has changed dramatically over centuries. Often descended from morally suspect theatrical clans, eighteenth- and nineteenth-century female dancers occupied a liminal status in a social system that at once admired them, used them, and turned its back on them. Ballerinas like Dumilâtre embodied the contradictions of their eras. They often wielded more autonomy than did most of their female contemporaries, but their livelihoods were also often entirely contingent on the support of male lovers. In late nineteenth-century Russia, Karsavina was raised in the Imperial Ballet School as a servant of the tsar; as such, though, she was more educated and better provided for than many other young women of her class. There was a seismic shift in the twentieth century, when (typically) only young women of upper-middle-class families could be given access to dance training. These women were educated and often faced the confusing stricture that, while their families might permit them to dabble in dance, it was never intended that they should perform onstage. And all faced pressures to combine family expectations and livelihoods, frequently juggling the demands of family and careers.

Baccelli and Dumilâtre were born into theatrical families and thus occupied a position outside polite society. However, both were trained in their profession and educated; they were not "lower class" in the accepted definition of the term. They were working women of the theater who depended to some degree on male patrons. These ballerinas thus occupied a social caste that was permeable and highly insecure; as successful dancers and beautiful women, Baccelli and Dumilâtre were able to support their livelihoods, in part, because they filled a desirable niche as lovers to men of the leisure classes. Had the two women been less successful or not quite as beautiful, they might have lost their status as star dancers and fallen into the ranks of the anonymous hordes of working but impoverished female dancers.

That Tamara Karsavina was a luminary in the Diaghilev Ballets Russes is only part of the true picture of her life as a working artist. She was also a teacher, a writer, and a staunch support to the developing British ballet in the early to middle decades of the twentieth century. In spite of her *almost* legendary fame, important aspects of her life and career remain under-recognized. While Karsavina herself, like Baccelli and Dumilâtre, emerged from a family of theater folk, she was brought up to reside in that ambiguous social caste between the nobility and the peasant. Raised as an artist, she received an exceptionally fine education and was trained to be disciplined and attentive to her art. Yet, her life as a child in the Theatre School of the Imperial Russian Ballet was austere and heavily circumscribed, and she was not granted many of the social freedoms Baccelli and Dumilâtre would have known as "loose" women of the stage. Emerging in the twentieth century as a young star of the Diaghilev Ballets Russes, Karsavina was treated as an artist and an educated woman of the world. However, her acknowledged sensibility and artistic refinement did not guarantee there would always be food on her table, and many times during her life Karsavina would find herself dancing to support her home and family.

Though Moira Shearer might have been the first to acknowledge that she was not Margot Fonteyn, the Scottish ballerina built a considerable reputation. But what is less recognized is that her career trajectory ran into significant tensions in twentieth-century ballet. Shearer crossed another boundary, that between ballet as a so-called high art form and the world of film, seen sometimes as a tawdry popular entertainment. Through her appearances in several well-known films, she encountered the mid-twentieth-century British agenda that ballet should be treated as high art and the decision by significant dancers, funders, and critics that ballet should lay claim to its own canon of historically established masterpieces.[2] In hindsight, Shearer and others believed this decision to appear in films may have "sullied" her in the eyes of Ninette de Valois, the resolute and pragmatic director of the Vic-Wells Ballet. That these two women differed in their accounts of events, and that they apparently did not agree on many points, was only one part of Shearer's working life as a ballerina. However, the tensions of her professional life, as well as the very strong pull of motherhood and family, led to what seems to have been her premature retirement from ballet.

Catherine Kerr, like the choreographer for whom she worked, is a woman of quiet determination and incisive intelligence. However, her forcefulness on stage and her tremendous contribution to the work of Merce Cunningham are less than fully recognized, for the company as a whole maintains a policy of no-star anonymity. Nevertheless, her bodily presence in the dances that Cunningham made for her remains in the roles today danced by younger women. The shape of her body—the physicality with which she invested her dance—helped to create the look of the Cunningham repertory in the dances of the 1970s and 1980s.

Each woman in this account had her subjective story and bore her own private tensions, conflicts, and difficulties, and each knew her personal moments of triumph or joy. But issues of class, education, social status, training modalities, ambition, jealousy, sexuality, and motherhood remained constant. Still elusive are these underlying questions: Why do women choose to dance in the first place? Once inside the ballet studio, why do they choose to stick to dance in spite of all its privations and difficulties? I cannot conclusively answer these questions, of course; I can only imagine that each woman would echo Vicky Page and Lermontov in their initial conversation in *The Red Shoes: I don't know exactly why, but I must.*

NOTES

INTRODUCTION

1. Royer, *Histoire de l'Opéra*, 170.
2. Koritz, *Gendering Bodies/Performing Art*, 1.
3. The writer Toni Bentley is one exception. As a dancer in the corps of New York City Ballet, Bentley kept a journal for a time. See her book *Winter Season.*
4. Koritz, *Gendering Bodies/Performing Art*, 1.
5. Banes, *Dancing Women*, 2.
6. Perrot, *From the Fires of Revolution*, 4.
7. Morrison, "The Site of Memory," 302.
8. Foreman, *Georgiana Duchess of Devonshire*, xiii. The historian Arlette Farge describes a similar process: "Emotion. The word is out! It is a word which is almost taboo for anyone who professes to be a student of social matters. . . . [But emotion] is one of the main supports for the process of research and understanding; and it is through the breach opened up between oneself and the object under consideration that enquiry enters in." Farge, *Fragile Lives*, 3–4.
9. Gaddis, *Landscape of History*, 45–46.

CHAPTER 1: GIOVANNA BACCELLI

1. Elizabeth Einberg documents the history of the portrait: "Painted for John Frederick Sackville, 3rd Duke of Dorset; remained at Knole, Sevenoaks, until 1890, when sold privately to S. Cunliffe-Lister (later Lord Masham); purchased from the Trustees of the Swinton Settled Estates, via Christie, Manson & Woods Ltd, 1975, with a

contribution from the Friends of the Tate Gallery." Einberg, *Gainsborough's Giovanna Baccelli*, 30.

2. Wall text accompanying the portrait at Tate Britain, London.

3. Postle, "'Modern Apelles,'" 180–97.

4. Einberg, *Gainsborough's Giovanna Baccelli*, 14.

5. Guest, *Ballet of the Enlightenment*, 205.

6. Ivor Guest calls her Janette. Guest, "Italian Lady," 79. According to Highfill, Burnim, and Langhans, she was sometimes known as Gianett. Highfill, Burnim, and Langhans, *Biographical Dictionary*, 190.

7. See Dalla Valle, "La fama vien danzando," regarding Baccelli's fluency in French. As for her abilities with the English language, Einberg quotes a letter from Baccelli to George Nassau, third Earl Cowper: "Knole, 12 August 1789 . . . Isn't life good in Florence my Lord? But England is more beautiful than ever, and I am sure that when you return to your native shore, you will agree that one can enjoy life in this Country too." Einberg, *Gainsborough's Giovanna Baccelli*, 13.

8. Twenty-one is fairly late for a modern-day ballet dancer to begin her career; it would seem to be very late for an eighteenth-century dancer to do so. Her probable age at her first London appearance suggests that Baccelli may well have performed elsewhere before going to London. There are accounts of performances by fairly young children. The daughters of Monsieur and Madame Simonet, for example, performed on various occasions at ages as young as six, seven, and eight. The well-known German ballerina Anne Heinel was seen dancing in Paris when she was sixteen. The young prodigy Auguste Vestris was celebrated for his first appearance at the age of twelve. See individual entries in Highfill, Burnim, and Langhans, *Biographical Dictionary*.

9. See Winter, *The Theatre of Marvels*, 108–9.

10. Guest, *Ballet of the Enlightenment*, 25. Marie Sallé (1707–56) was another such classically trained ballerina whose family was a band of theatrical itinerants. Parmenia Migel reports that one of Sallé's uncles was a famous tumbler-harlequin-comedian who directed a troupe of roving performers, which included a family member who was a clown and another who was an acrobat. See Migel, *The Ballerinas*, 16.

11. Guest, *Ballet of the Enlightenment*, 25.

12. V. Sackville-West, *Knole and the Sackvilles*, 189.

13. Hallet, "Reynolds, Celebrity and the Exhibition Space," 37.

14. Dorset's mistresses included Nancy Parsons, Mrs. Elizabeth Armistead, Lady Betty Hamilton, Lady Elizabeth Foster, and, according to some, Georgiana, Duchess of Devonshire. V. Sackville-West, *Knole and the Sackvilles*, 178–80.

15. Today, avid cricket players in Sevenoaks are proud that because of the duke's love for the game, their small town has achieved recognition in histories of the sport. In his description of Knole written for the National Trust, Robert Sackville writes: "At Knole [the duke] employed a small squad of professional cricketers, including the bowler 'Lumpy' Stevens, whose prowess was partly responsible for the introduction of the third stump. In the early days of cricket, the wicket consisted of only two stumps; however, in a match between Hambledon and Kent in 1775, Lumpy bowled several balls in succession straight through his opponent's wicket. When Hambledon played England at Sevenoaks in 1777, Vine ground, three stumps were used for the first time." R. Sackville-West, *Knole, Kent*, 83.

16. Ibid.

17. Hallet, "Reynolds, Celebrity and the Exhibition Space," 35 (quote).

18. In the 1780s, British newspapers started to have better-informed and more accurate writing about dance. Some press accounts were straightforward reviews, but others were "bought" by rival stars. See Price, Milhous, and Hume, *Italian Opera*, 443.

19. Quoted in Highfill, Burnim, and Langhans, *Biographical Dictionary*, 192.

20. Ibid., 191

21. But such circumstances were not always reported. The *Morning Herald* of June 1, 1781, gave an account of the theatrical mayhem that ensued when news of Baccelli's illness reached the expectant audience by word of mouth:

> A Fracas happened last night at the King's Theatre, on account of the first Ballet not being danced as advertised. The sober part of the audience took it good naturedly, a whisper having gone round, that M. Bacelli [*sic*] was indisposed, and unable to execute her parts in the first and last dances, which was the real fact. But some malcontents in the upper regions having signified very vociferously their displeasure, Mr. Crawford stept forward with the two Vestris to make a proper apology. The cry of hear him was for some time drowned in the noisy sound of sticks, groans, and hisses; he was at last permitted to inform them, that Baccelli's indisposition was the the [*sic*] cause of their disappointment.—This would certainly have produced the desired effect, had not one of the company stood up as the confessed ringleader of the whole party of dissatisfied spectators; who, with clinched [*sic*] fists, gnashing of teeth, and high sounding imprecations kept up the ball for some time; 'till the manager coming forth once more, assured the audience that their desire would be complied with. All were now satisfied, except the person alluded to, who seem'd galled at the reconciliation likely to take place: nay, when the wish'd-for dancers appeared, and were received with the loudest applause, the clamorous gentleman continued to spit his venom, which indeed was lavished to no other purpose, than to convince his neighbours that (being himself of the profession) envy alone had excited his spleen.

22. Guest, "Italian Lady," 85.

23. John Chapman asserts that Gardel held a "central position in ballet history, for his ballets were models of excellence," and his "teaching was respected by ballet 'giants' such as Noverre, Blasis and Bournonville." Chapman, "Forgotten Giant," 3.

24. Foreman, *Georgiana Duchess of Devonshire*, 233.

25. Einberg, *Gainsborough's Giovanna Baccelli*, 9–10.

26. Quoted, Walpole, *Correspondences*, vol. 43, 291n.

27. Einberg, *Gainsborough's Giovanna Baccelli*, 10.

28. Ibid., 15.

29. Ibid.

30. Chapman, "Auguste Vestris and the Expansion of Technique," 1.

31. Ibid., 11.

32. Ibid., 12.

33. Ibid., 14.

34. Gallini became the proprietor of the theater, serving from 1785 to 1789. Also teaching and composing dances at the King's Theatre during Baccelli's career were

Simon Slingsby, Louis Simonet, and Charles Le Picq. Ivor Guest suggests that when Pierre Gardel arrived in London in the early 1780s, Baccelli probably seized the opportunity to train with him as well. Guest, *Ballet of the Enlightenment*, 205.

35. Gallini, *Treatise*, 51.

36. The beating on the ground was similar to a modern-day *battement frappé*. The beaten jump was like an *entrechat*. Today the form in which the leg is lifted might be called a *battement dégagé* (low level) or a *grand battement* (at hip height or above).

37. Magri, *Theoretical and Practical Treatise*, 73. The *ballerino* is comparable to the *danseur noble* in the French categorization. Magri distinguishes the three types of dancers in Italian terminology: the noble *ballerini*, the broader and more vivacious *mezzo carattere*, and the virtuosic, even acrobatic *grotesco*.

38. Ibid.

39. See the discussion in Magri, "Of the Equilibrium of the Body," chapter 4 in his *Theoretical and Practical Treatise*.

40. Judging from recorded images (including Gainsborough's portrait of Baccelli), this turnout would have been greater than that practiced in the ballroom, but would not have reached the 180 degrees that would become the ideal later. The introduction of the pointe shoe and the greater emphasis on pointe work early in the nineteenth century were two of the significant milestones in the greater use of turnout.

41. Magri, *Theoretical and Practical Treatise*, 56.

42. In the chapter entitled "Of the Equilibrium of the Body" (ibid., 56–57), Magri described six ways of attaining balance:

> I. Naturally supporting the body on both feet with the torso very straight so that if a plumb line were hung from the *sternum* or intercostal bone . . . that is, the bone of the thorax to which the ribs are attached, the line would fall plumb in the centre of that space between the feet.
>
> II. The body is balanced on the balls of both feet with the same symmetry.
>
> III. On the sole of one foot, lightly touching the ground with only the tip of the other and then it is necessary to slightly incline the body to the side of the foot which is flat on the ground, because otherwise it would be impossible to achieve just equilibrium, since the two feet do not form an equal base as before.
>
> IV. With one foot in the air, and the whole body supported on the sole of the other.
>
> V. On the ball of one foot, holding the other in the air.
>
> VI. Sustaining the body over both heels, without the rest of the foot touching the ground, and here the body will be perpendicular as in the first equilibrium.

43. Noverre, *Letters on Dancing*, 119.

44. Lynham, *Chevalier Noverre*, 127.

45. Noverre, *Letters on Dancing*, 78.

46. Noverre, *Letters on Dancing*, 86–87.

47. For further information on the relationship between fashion and theatrical dress, please see Edmund Fairfax's very helpful appendix entitled "Remarks on Costume," in his *Styles of Eighteenth-Century Ballet*.

48. Davenport, *Book of Costume*, 655.

49. Cohen, *Art, Dance, and the Body*, 37–38.

50. Lynham, *Chevalier Noverre*, 120.

51. Ibid., 120–21.

52. The growth in audiences also affected the architecture of the opera houses, a phenomenon described by Margarete Baur-Heinhold in *The Baroque Theatre*. "It is a commonly held opinion," she writes,

> that the introduction of galleries in theatres was entirely due to the rigid social stratification of the seventeenth and eighteenth centuries, that they were designed to uphold the class distinctions whose immutability was an essential factor of the age of Absolutism. But this is not necessarily the only explanation. Ever greater numbers of people wanting to go to the theatres had to be accommodated in buildings on the limited sites available in the centre of old cities. The only possible direction of expansion was upwards, which necessarily meant building tiers of galleries. Another factor is acoustic: the horsehoe shape of theatre is the most favourable to the clarity of musical sounds, particularly the human voice singing *pianissimo* (163).

53. In her *Dance in the Shadow of the Guillotine*, Judith Chazin-Bennahum describes the byzantine system of regulations and privileges. See chapter 3, "Theatres in Paris, or the Beset Stage," 20–26.

54. Lynham, *Chevalier Noverre*, 82.

55. Ibid., 84–85.

56. Guest, *Ballet of the Enlightenment*, 179.

57. Quoted in Price, Milhous, and Hume, *Italian Opera*, 180.

58. Guest, *Ballet of the Enlightenment*, 205–6.

59. Ibid., 206n. For further discussion of the beginnings of *pointe* work, see Hammond, "Searching for the Sylph."

60. For further information on the range of dance qualities involved in each of the four styles of ballet, see Fairfax, *Styles of Eighteenth-Century Ballet*.

61. Fairfax, *Styles of Eighteenth-Century Ballet*, 94.

62. Quoted, ibid., 104.

63. Ibid., 103.

64. See Duplain, "Guimard."

65. Duplain (ibid.) describes the emotional shift that takes place in this scene:

> Ces souris enfantins, l'ame de la gaité;
> Et ces gestes, l'éclair de la naïveté.
> Mais quel contraste affreux! Déese trop crédule,
> Elle échappe à l'acier & le poison circule.
> Son bras ne soutient plus la forme des cerceaux;
> Son oeil s'appésantit, ses pas sont inégaux;
> Sur son front se répand une pâleur extrême;
> Elle gémit, s'ignore & se cherche elle-même.
> Chaque fibre affaiblie exprime un sentiment,
> Et peint dans tout son corps l'anéantissement.

66. The scene in which Colas comes across the disguised Ninette at court is described in terms of facial expression and gesture:

La Comtesse parâit, rit de ton peu d'usage.
Tu pinces ton fichu, caresses ton corsage,
Danses très pesamment, ou, telle qu'un éclair,
Entasses des coulés affectes le bel air,
Et mêles ce croquis de ruses si nouvelles,
Qu'il fixe Cupidon & lui coupe les aîles.
Espiègle de Momus tu lutines Colas,
Qui, sous ton voile heureux, ne te reconnaît pas.
Il refuse tes dons. . . . Séduisante imposture,
Quelle pâleur s'oppose au cours de la nature!
Simulacre de mort, adorable langueur,
Suspend. . . . Colas lui-même est bientôt sans vigueur.
Tu renais cependant & je vois sur ta bouche
Un souris délicat qui pénètre & qui touche.

67. For an illustration of this work, see Burnim and Highfill, *John Bell*, #86.

68. Thornwaite worked during the years 1771–95.

69. Price, Milhous, and Hume write that "Noverre chose to feature Mme. Simonet where reputation might suggest that Mlle Baccelli or Mlle Théodore would take precedence." According to these writers, Simonet was the best actress of the three and Noverre treated her as "the ranking ballerina of the company, a prominence she was never again to enjoy." Price, Milhous, and Hume, *Italian Opera*, 463.

70. Guest, "Italian Lady," 82.

71. For a discussion of this incident, see Guest, "Italian Lady," 78–85.

72. The January 21, 1789, *Gazzetta* refers to her as "la vigorasa e leggiadrissima Mad. Baccelli." The February 7 account declares, "E' sè conosciuto, ammirato, e d'alte comuni lodi compensato il somme merito della veramente celebre Signora Bacelli." My thanks to Gino Biondini and Bettina Capello for translations from the Italian, here and below.

73. The account of January 28, 1789, reads:

Senza fare un esame analittico all'invenzione del Sig. Clerico; ma parlando soltanto dell'arte con cui ha posto in varj ben disegnati movimenti le sue figure e del ballabile che vi ha trat o tratto intodotto per lunga pantomima, confessare si deve che fu il suo lavoro molto studiato, faticoso, e degno del felice destino che compensò il suoi sudori. Senza pregiudizio del sno merito accordare però si deve, ch'hanno molto contribuito a metterlo nella più bella sua vista delle scene superbe, un vestíario ricco e magnifico, decorazioni di molta spesa, ed assai più un'abilissime Compagnia danzatrice, particolamente per l'inimitabile Mad. Baccelli il cui valor e superiore a ogni elogi, e per il leggiadrissimo Sig. Angiolini. Questa Coppia dopo avere nel primo Ballo esegiuta colla maggior bravura la sua parte, formò le delizie del secondo con un Pas-de-deux si gentile, ben ideato eseguito con tanta esatezza, d'una musica si parlante, d'un [caraterre ?] nella sua semplicità cosi amabile. da meritar ogni sera un pierno Teatro s'altro non fosse stato da veder che quello. Il sommo pregio di Mad. Baccelli è d'eseguire in Ballo le più difficili operazioni con una disinvoltura, e una sicurezza che le far parer facili celandone la fatica. Questa è l'art e dell'arte si rara nel a sua professione, che tanto cara la rende al Pubblico suo ammiratore, e fa portar nelle colorate cocardes a tante e tante per sone il segno d'un partito ch'onora il merito eccelso.

74. The passage, from a *Gazzetta* article of January 14, 1789, reads: "l'inimitabile Mad. Baccelli forma la delizia del gusto piu raffinato coll'esattezza, la leggiadria, la precisione, e la forza ond'eseguite sono le belle sue operazioni in quel mezzo nobil caractere, nel qual Ella è singolare ed eccellente."

75. The article reads:

Il genio instancabile della celebre Mad. Baccelli unito al più onesto zelo de 'vantaggy dell'Impresa a cui serve, inventar le fece un pezzo ballabile, che in Franca chiamerebbesi un Pot-Pourri, e trà noi può dirsi un capriccio adattato agli ultimi giorni di Carnovale, in cui ella eseguira in Ballo certe moderne canzonette popolari le cui Arie facili cantate son per le strade. La prodigiosa abilità di questa famosa Ballerina che supera qualanque difficoltà, e sà piegarsi a tutti i modi diversi le farà ottenere anche in questo un meritato pienissimo applauso, mosso dall ammirazione dal diletto, e da una certa giocondità, ch'ella sparge colle grzie ed il brio, ch'accompagna, no le difficili sue operazioni, le quali prendono dalla sua franchezza, e somma perizia nell'arte, un aria d'agevole efecuzione. *Gazzetta Urbana Venetia,* February 18, 1789.

76. See Fairfax, *Styles of Eighteenth-Century Ballet,* chapter 6.

77. The *Gazzetta Urbana Venetia* for February 21, 1789, reports:

Un accidente fatale non permise, che la celebre Madama Bacelli potesse eseguire la giocosa danza da lei ideata, nella sera dello scorso Mercordì. L'abilissimo suo compagno Signor Angiolini, saltando trà le scene, prima che cominciasse il Ballo, per iscaldarsi le gambe com'è costume de Ballerini, trovò sventuratamente cadendo la punta d'un chiodo, che gli si conficcò nel dito grosso d'un piede, onde fu in necessità di pronta assistenza chirugica, e di riposo.

Spargendosi la trista nuova di bocca in bocca ricevè il solito aumento. Asserivano alcuni, che non averebbe potuto ballare mai più, altri più discreti nel loro rammarico, che sarebbe guarito, ma non poteva certamente essere in istato d'adoperar i piedi in queste ultime recite dell'opera.

Sentiamo però con sodisfazione, che questa sera potrà egli agire nel corpo de'Balli, ed eseguire il nuovo Pas de deux colla volorosissima, e non mai lodata quanto n'è degna, sua compagna.

78. Lowe, *La Serenissima,* 22.

79. Ibid., 64–65. Unlike dancers, actresses were reputed to be highly virtuous family women. They were customarily invited to family dinners by theater-goers of all social classes.

80. Andrieux, *Daily Life in Venice,* 189.

81. Price, Milhous, and Hume, *Italian Opera,* 441.

82. Adelaide Simonet was married to Louis Simonet and they had three daughters: Leonora, Rosine, and Theresa. Louis Simonet, a dancer, ballet master, violinist, and teacher, continued to dance at the King's Theatre until 1788 and served as a ballet master until about 1791. Geltruda Rossi was the mistress (and later, possibly, the wife) of the

ballet master Charles Le Picq, and both danced at the King's Theatre during Baccelli's years there. While it is not possible to determine when Rossi and Le Picq began their liaison, it is known that they were frequent dance partners. By 1785–86 they both had left the King's Theatre; Charles Le Picq reportedly went to Russia as a dance master in about 1786, with a "new" wife named Gertrude[?] Rossi. See individual entries in Highfill, Burnhim, and Langhans, *Biographical Dictionary.*

CHAPTER 2: ADÈLE DUMILÂTRE

1. Pierre-Jules-Théophile Gautier was born in Tarbes, in the south of France, on August 31, 1811.

2. Gautier, *Gautier on Dance,* 99.

3. Among many examples are the "sisters" Indiana and Noun in George Sand's 1832 novel *Indiana.* Marilyn Yalom, in her introduction to the 1993 Signet Classic edition of the novel, has this to say about the two women's relationship:

> Having nursed at the same breast, they are spiritual sisters, despite the difference in their social positions. Each is endowed with the physical attributes deemed appropriate to her social station: Noun is tall, strong, healthy, and passionate, whereas Indiana is pale and frail and, implicitly, less hot-blooded than the true Creole. Individually they are stereotypes of their respective classes; together they constitute a whole person who has been fragmented by social proscriptions. Indiana's compelling sense of sisterhood with Noun far exceeds the conventional bonds between mistress and confidante: it suggests the union of a "respectable" woman and what Jung would have called her "shadow" self (xi–xii).

4. Lisa Arkin and Marian Smith discuss the under-recognized importance of folk dance, often called national or character dance, in the romantic ballet. See their "National Dance in the Romantic Ballet," in Garafola, *Rethinking the Sylph,* 11–68.

5. Gautier, review, "La Tarentulle," in *Gautier on Dance,* 70.

6. Second, *Les petits mystères de l'Opéra,* 114.

7. *Bulletin Théâtral,* March 30, 1841, reports Dumilâtre's debut in the role made famous by Marie Taglioni in 1832: "Cette jeune et jolie danseuse se recommande par beaucoup de grâce; quelquefois même, elle trouve des élans subits, elle atteint un certain degré de noblesse et de vigueur."

8. Royer, *Histoire de l'Opéra,* 170.

9. Lumley, *Reminiscences of the Opera,* 64.

10. Guest, *Jules Perrot,* 93.

11. The print I saw was published in London by J. Mitchell on April 23, 1843. It is archived at the Harvard Theatrical Collection.

12. Guest, *Ballet of the Second Empire,* 36–37.

13. Although Castil-Blaze reports that it was the elder of the two sisters (Sophie) who married del Castillo, it was in fact the younger, Adèle.

14. Guest, *Ballet of the Second Empire,* 37.

15. Quoted, ibid., 68.

16. Garafola, *Rethinking the Sylph* 4.

17. "Pour l'empêcher de tomber, lorsqu'elle exécute des poses trop penchées ou de périlleuses pirouettes." Royer, *Histoire de l'Opéra*, 169.

18. Castil-Blaze, *L'Académie impériale de musique*, 273.

19. Garafola, "The Travesty Dancer in Nineteenth-Century Ballet," 35.

20. Ibid., 39.

21. Gautier, *Gautier on Dance*, 35.

22. Quoted in Chapman, "Jules Janin," 231–32.

23. Notably, in his own post as dancing master at the Royal Theatre of Copenhagen, Bournonville managed to maintain the status of male dancers. Knud Arne Jürgensen writes, "With courage and persistence Bournonville championed the male dancer in an era of female adulation and brought natural warmth and humanity to the often exaggeratedly mysterious atomsphere of Romantic ballet." Jürgensen, *The Bournonville Tradition*, 142. However, until the arrival of the Diaghilev Ballets Russes in Paris in the early twentieth century, male dancers had virtually disappeared from the ballet in the rest of western Europe. See the discussion in Garafola, *Diaghilev's Ballets Russes.*

24. Bournonville, *Letters on Dance and Choreography.* 37.

25. Ibid.

26. *The Raft of the Medusa* (1819), an emblematic work in Romantic art, was painted by Théodore Géricault (1791–1824). Victor Hugo's 1830 tragedy *Hernani* was the basis for Verdi's opera *Ernani.* In her introduction to Gautier's *Mademoiselle de Maupin,* Joanna Richardson writes, "On 25 February 1830, wearing a flamboyant and now legendary pink doublet, Gautier joined Hugo's supporters at the Théâtre-Français. It was the first night of *Hernani:* the night that was to determine the prestige—one might almost say the supremacy—of the new Romantic literature. It was the decisive encounter between traditional and progressive, past and future, Classicism and Romanticism." Gautier, *Mademoiselle de Maupin,* 6.

27. J.-G. Prod'homme in *L'Opéra (1669–1925)* lists some of the era's most famous ballet masters and the periods of their activity. These include: Coralli, 1802–50; Decombe, known as Albert, 1803–09, 1817–31; Taglioni, 1806–?; Mérante, 1808–33; Paul, 1813–32; Elie, 1810–17; Coulon, 182?–1849; Montessu, 1817–30; Barrez, 1821–44; Théodore, 1827–47; Paul Taglioni, 1827–; Coralli fils, 1831–46; Albert fils, 1836–?; Petipa, 1839–50; Mabille, 1836–50; Mazilier, 1830–68; and Saint-Léon, 1846–53, 1855.

28. For further information see Hammond, "Searching for the Sylph."

29. Most prominent among these scholars are Knud Arne Jürgensen, Erik Ashengreen, and Patricia N. McAndrew.

30. Bournonville, *New Year's Gift,* 7.

31. Quoted in Jürgensen, *Bournonville Tradition,* 34–35.

32. Ibid., 37.

33. Bournonville, *New Year's Gift,* 10.

34. Gautier, *Histoire de l'art dramatique,* 42.

35. Chapman, "Jules Janin," 199.

36. For an overview, see Cranston, *Romantic Movement.*

37. Gautier, *Maupin,* 19.

38. Ibid., 39.

39. Cranston, *Romantic Movement,* 93.

40. See, for instance, the discussion in Winter, *Theatre of Marvels.*

41. Tragically, gas lighting also led to the premature and painful deaths by fire of many gauze-clad *danseuses.* For an account of one example, see Guest, *Victorian Ballet Girl.*

42. See Smith, *Ballet and Opera in the Age of Giselle,* 3–18.

43. Quoted in Huckenpahler, "Confessions of an Opera Director," 73.

44. Thackeray, *Paris Sketch Book,* 9.

45. See the discussion of the *foyer* in Kahane, *Le foyer de la danse.*

46. Quoted in Second, *Petits mysteres de l'Opera,* 149–50.

47. See Robin-Challan, "Social Conditions of Ballet Dancers."

48. Ibid., 20.

49. Ibid., 21.

50. Ibid.

51. Baudelaire, *Painter of Modern Life,* 35.

52. McMillan, *France and Women,* 36.

53. Ibid., 39–40.

54. Bournonville, *Letters on Dance and Choreography,* 76.

55. Quoted in Maurice, *Histoire anecdotique de théatre,* 263.

56. Ibid., 267.

57. Beaumont, *Ballet Called Giselle,* 9.

58. Gautier, *Gautier on Dance,* 94.

59. Beaumont explains that Gautier took his inspiration for the ballet not only from the work of Heinrich Heine, but also from Victor Hugo's poem "Fantômes," in which a young woman, passionate about dance, dies of overheated excitement after leaving ballroom in cold dawn. One line says, "Elle aimait trop le bal, c'est ce qui l'a tuée." At first, Beaumont writes, Gautier envisioned a mimed depiction of Hugo's poem. He imagined the young girl dancing at a ball that was also attended by the icy cold queen of the wilis. According to Beaumont, "The Queen of the Wilis would have touched the floor with her magic wand to fill the dancers' feet with an insatiable desire for contredanses, waltzes, galops, and mazurkas. The advent of the lords and ladies would have made them fly away like so many vague shadows. Giselle, having danced all that evening, excited by the magic floor and the desire to keep her lover from inviting other women to dance, would have been suprised by the cold dawn like the young Spanish girl [of Hugo's poem], and the pale Queen of the Wilis, invisible to all, would have laid her icy hand on her heart." Unable to turn this idea into a ballet, however, Gautier turned to Saint-Georges to create a dramatic and stage-worthy scenario. Beaumont, *Ballet Called Giselle,* 20.

60. Gautier, *Gautier on Dance,* 98–99.

61. Quoted in Chapman, "Jules Janin," 235.

62. Ibid., 238.

63. Arkin and Smith, "National Dance in the Romantic Ballet," 48. For discussion of the entire ballet, see also Smith, *Ballet and Opera in the Age of Giselle.*

64. Quoted in Chapman, "Jules Janin," 241.

65. Guest, *Romantic Ballet in Paris,* 226–27.

66. Gerken, "Chambermaids for Hire," 21

67. Gautier, *Gautier on Dance,* 124.

68. Such musical pastiches were common, however, and the unevenness of the score can hardly have been a surprise.

69. Gautier, *Gautier on Dance,* 125.

70. These plates are housed at the Harvard Theatrical Collection.

71. In the ballet's original *livret* the name is written "Plumket."

72. Gautier, *Gautier on Dance,* 128.

73. Ibid.

74. Ibid.

75. A print available in the Harvard Theatrical Collection bears no evident date or publication information. This print is published in Guest, *Gallery of Romantic Ballet,* plate 55.

76. Binney, *Glories of the Romantic Ballet,* 85.

77. Letter from the Salem Collection at Harvard Theatrical Collection, MS 415. The choreographer was Arthur Saint-Léon.

78. See Binney, *Glories of the Romantic Ballet,* 100, plates 77A and 77B.

79. Dunning, "In 'Giselle,' the Acting Informs the Dance," comments on the "womanly Myrtha" of Corella and the "majestic" dancing of Wiles.

80. Hering, "Dancing the Classics."

81. Kisselgoff, "Dance of Remorse and Regeneration."

CHAPTER 3: TAMARA KARSAVINA

1. Kyasht recalls: "One of my greatest friends at the Imperial Ballet School was Tamara Karsavina, who was destined to make her name as a *Première Danseuse.* We played together and we took our punishments together, for both of us were mischievous children and full of high spirits, although in justice to Tamara I must admit that I was usually the ring-leader in our pranks, while she was an obedient lieutenant." Kyasht, *Romantic Recollections,* 21.

2. In her 1975 book *Diaghilev Observed by Critics,* Nesta McDonald explains that Barrie's original play was to feature Lydia Lopokova. But Lopokova disappeared from the scene for a time, and Barrie met, and was charmed by, Karsavina. Because Karsavina's English was not as fluent as Lopokova's, Barrie had the idea of revising the play to feature a ballerina who would dance her part instead of speaking her lines. Karsavina, writes McDonald, "devised her own language of mime for the part of 'Karissima of the Ballet'" (256–57).

3. Bruce, *Thirty Dozen Moons,* 104.

4. Garafola, *Diaghilev's Ballets Russes,* 227.

5. Karsavina, *Theatre Street,* 19.

6. Fokine wrote: "On entering the school I was placed in the class of Karsavin, and for the first six months was limited to doing bar work. The following half year I began to work in the center, which really amounted to doing the same exercises . . . no longer holding on to the bar, but standing in the middle of the floor. Nowadays the slow tempo and the monotony of these lessons seem amazing to me. Actually, however, this patient, slow work trained my legs so that for the rest of my life I was preserved from

the handicaps which a dancer encounters if he begins his studies later in life or proceeds too rapidly to the study of a more interesting phase of the dance without preparing a proper foundation for it." Fokine, *Memoirs*, 24.

7. Karsavina, *Theatre Street*, 25.

8. Ibid.

9. Ibid., 26.

10. Ibid., 27.

11. Ibid., 36.

12. Ibid., 58.

13. Ibid., 47.

14. Roslavleva, *Era of the Russian Ballet*, 109.

15. Ibid., 111.

16. Karsavina, *Theatre Street*, 132.

17. Kschessinska, *Dancing in Petersburg*, 24.

18. Karsavina, *Theatre Street*, 68. If in writing these memoirs the irony of this situation occurred to her, Karsavina never mentioned it; a few decades later, she would be the foreign star bringing Russian ballet to the West. Many non-Russian dancers would change their names to sound Russian so as to be taken seriously by European and American audiences.

19. Ibid.

20. Kschessinska, *Dancing in Petersburg*, 45.

21. Karsavina, *Theatre Street*, 69.

22. Ibid., 70.

23. Ibid., 78–79.

24. Ibid., 107.

25. Ibid., 98.

26. Ibid., 102.

27. Ibid., 111.

28. Scholl writes, "Imperial patronage enabled the Russian ballet to prosper in the late nineteenth century, at a time when ballet in Western Europe was in decline, but the ballet suffered from its reputation as an aristocratic bauble." Scholl, *From Petipa to Balanchine*, 14.

29. Lincoln, *Sunlight at Midnight*, 105.

30. Benois, *Memoirs*, 30.

31. Ibid., 39–40.

32. Garafola, *Diaghilev's Ballets Russes*, 163.

33. Lincoln, *The Romanovs*, 607.

34. Banes, *Dancing Women*, 64.

35. Karsavina, *Theatre Street*, 124.

36. Ibid., 124–25.

37. Kschessinska, *Dancing in Petersburg*, 87–88.

38. Karsavina, *Theatre Street*, 135.

39. Ibid.

40. Ibid., 136.

41. Ibid., 145.

42. Ibid., 148–49.

43. Garafola, *Diaghilev's Ballets Russes*, 191.

44. Karsavina, *Theatre Street*, 179.

45. Lydia Kyasht also studied with Madame Sokolva. She recalled, "She was a remarkable woman altogether, and had enjoyed the unique position of having been a platonic favourite of the Tsar Alexander the Second. So highly indeed did this Emperor esteem her, that he even granted her permission to wed a naval officer. This action roused considerable comment in St. Petersburg, as it was a generally accepted rule that no dancers of the Imperial Ballet School were allowed to wed either an officer of the Imperial Navy or of the Imperial Army, unless the reigning Tsar chose to grant a special dispensation in their favour, and it was seldom that any Emperor exercised this Imperial prerogative." Kyasht, *Romantic Recollections*, 47–48.

46. Karsavina, *Theatre Street*, 181.

47. Ibid., 181–82.

48. Ibid., 150.

49. Roslavleva, *Era of the Russian Ballet*, 89 (quote).

50. Ibid., 85.

51. Scholl, *From Petipa to Balanchine*, 3.

52. Roslavleva, *Era of the Russian Ballet*, 86 (quotes). As Scholl sums up Petipa's vast output, "only six of the full-length ballets choreographed by Petipa are still performed. Three of these date from the last phase of Petipa's career: *Sleeping Beauty* (1890), *Swan Lake* (1895), and *Raymonda* (1898). These ballets, to music of Pyotr Tchaikovsky and Aleksandr Glazunov, are Petipa's best-known works. Standards of the international repertory, they have come down to us in reasonably authentic versions. The ballets that survive from the first decades of Petipa's work in Russia—*Le Corsaire* (1863), *Don Quixote* (1869), *La Bayadère* (1877)—have suffered infrequent, less faithful revivals." Scholl, *From Petipa to Balanchine*, 4.

53. Roslavleva, *Era of the Russian Ballet*, 86 (quotes). *Ballabili* is an Italian word introduced into French and referring to a dance for a large number of dancers.

54. Scholl, *From Petipa to Balanchine*, 8–9.

55. Garafola, *Diaghilev's Ballets Russes*, 8.

56. Quoted, ibid.

57. Ibid.

58. Ibid., 9.

59. Lincoln, *The Romanovs*, 656.

60. Ibid., 657.

61. Garafola, *Diaghilev's Ballets Russes*, 4.

62. Karsavina, *Theatre Street*, 158.

63. Ibid., 159.

64. Garafola, *Diaghilev's Ballets Russes*, 5.

65. Ibid., 6.

66. Karsavina, *Theatre Street*, 169.

67. Fokine, *Memoirs*, 35.

68. Garafola, *Diaghilev's Ballets Russes*, 10.

69. Fokine, *Memoirs*, 51.

70. Karsavina, *Theatre Street*, 169.

71. Fokine, *Memoirs*, 130.

72. Drummond, *Speaking of Diaghilev*, 90–91.
73. Quoted, ibid., 90–91
74. Buckle, *In the Wake of Diaghilev*, 113.
75. Ibid., 113–14.
76. Ibid., 114.
77. Figes, *Natasha's Dance*, xxx.
78. Karsavina, *Theatre Street*, 189.
79. Garafola, *Diaghilev's Ballets Russes*, Preface, x.
80. Karsavina, *Theatre Street*, 192.
81. Ibid., 190.
82. Garafola, *Diaghilev's Ballets Russes*, 188.
83. Ibid., 165.
84. Karsavina, *Theatre Street*, 194.
85. Grigoriev, *Diaghilev Ballet*, 30.
86. Ibid., 31.
87. Karsavina, *Theatre Street*, 199.
88. Ibid., 204.
89. Ibid., 207.
90. Ibid., 205.
91. Garafola, "Reconfiguring the Sexes," 246.
92. Ibid. The men included Léonide Massine, Anton Dolin, Serge Lifar and some "lesser lights." See the discussion in Garafola, "Reconfiguring the Sexes."
93. Ibid., 249.
94. Haskell and Nouvel, *Diaghileff*, 208.
95. Lieven, *Birth of Ballets-Russes*, 147.
96. Haskell and Nouvel, *Diaghileff*, 208.
97. Lieven, *Birth of Ballets-Russes*, 159.
98. Grigoriev, *Diaghilev Ballet*, 39.
99. Karsavina, *Theatre Street*, 220.
100. Haskell and Nouvel, *Diaghileff*, 203.
101. Garafola, "Reconfiguring the Sexes," 251.
102. Karsavina, *Theatre Street*, 221–22.
103. Ibid., 221.
104. Ibid., 212.
105. Garafola, *Diaghilev's Ballets Russes*, 266.
106. Karsavina, "Why 'Ballet Russe' Could Not Survive Diaghileff," 53 (first, second, third quotes), 54 (fourth and fifth quotes).
107. Haskell, *Balletomania Then and Now*, 112.
108. Lieven, *Birth of Ballets-Russes*, 113.
109. Bruce, *Thirty Dozen Moons*, 29.
110. Ibid., 29–30.
111. Lieven, *Birth of Ballets-Russes*, 330–31.
112. Buckle, *In the Wake of Diaghilev*, 114.
113. Karsavina, *Theatre Street*, 265.
114. Ibid., 272.
115. Ibid., 271–73.

116. Bruce, *Thirty Dozen Moons*, 11.

117. Ibid., 28.

118. Ibid., 40.

119. Ibid., 47–48.

120. Quoted in Vaughan, *Frederick Ashton and His Ballets*, 59.

121. Clarke, *Six Great Dancers*, 124.

CHAPTER 4: MOIRA SHEARER

1. Christie, *Arrows of Desire*, 18.

2. The Vic-Wells later became the Sadler's Wells Ballet and then the Royal Ballet. The history of the company is amply documented. One contemporary account is that of A. H. Franks, who reports that by 1946 "the company which had during the war years quietly changed its name from the Vic-Wells Ballet to the Sadler's Wells Ballet, had installed itself at the Royal Opera House, Covent Garden, under the auspices of the Covent Garden Opera Trust." Franks, *Approach to the Ballet*, 140.

Established at the Royal Opera House, Covent Garden also initiated the founding of a second, touring company and necessitated a reorganization of the school. The Royal Ballet was instituted through Royal Charter on October 31, 1956, with the stated purpose "to promote and advance the art of the ballet and in association therewith the literary, musical and graphical arts and to foster public knowledge and appreciation of the same." Walker, *Ninette de Valois*, 282.

3. Quoted in Newman, *Striking a Balance*, 138.

4. Shearer, interview by Dale Harris, August 29, 1976, transcript, New York Public Library, 1–3. The Italian-born Enrico Cecchetti (1850–1928) arrived in St. Petersburg in 1887, taught at the Imperial Theatre School, and performed and taught for many decades with the Diaghilev Ballets Russes. He was a favored teacher of many illustrious dancers, including Pavlova. Cecchetti's codified system of classical training has been passed on to ballet teachers around the world.

5. Shearer, interview by Harris, transcript, 1–3. Nicolas Legat (1869–1937), born in St. Petersburg, was a *premier danseur* at the Maryinsky Theatre and for many years taught the Class of Perfection at the Imperial Theatre School. The last twelve years of his life were spent in London, where leading dancers sought him out to study with him.

6. Quoted in Newman, *Striking a Balance*, 118. Legat's wife, Nadine Nicolaeva, was herself a dancer and a sometime partner of Nicolas.

7. According to Frederick Ashton's biographer Julie Kavanaugh, this point was fiercely disputed by Ashton, who claimed that de Valois "absolutely abandoned us." His version of events is that at the outbreak of the war, he and the music director, Constant Lambert, reassembled the company, while de Valois went home to help her doctor husband with his medical clinic. Ashton and Lambert then organized to take the company on the road without orchestra but with two pianists. According to Ashton, "When Ninette saw it was going to work she came back and took the whole thing in her hands again." Kavanaugh, *Secret Muses*, 240–41.

8. De Valois, *Come Dance*, 144.

9. Craig-Raymond, "Career of Moira Shearer," 19.

10. Shearer, interview by Harris, transcript, 29–30.

11. Meredith Daneman writes that although *The Quest* was not a critical success, the debuts of seventeen-year-old Moira Shearer and fifteen-year-old Beryl Grey were seen as auspicious. Both young dancers suddenly appeared to challenge Margot Fonteyn's preeminent position. According to Daneman, Shearer's "film-star looks" and Grey's extraordinary technique caused Fonteyn to grapple with what was for her a new and shocking emotion: "envy." Daneman, *Margot Fonteyn*, 175–76.

12. Kavanaugh, *Secret Muses*, 372.

13. Quoted in Daneman, *Margot Fonteyn*, 224.

14. *Daily Express*, February 4, 1953.

15. Craig-Raymond, "Career of Moira Shearer," 3.

16. Eglevsky and Gregory, *Heritage of a Ballet Master*, 5.

17. In his memoirs, Michel Fokine explained the Imperial Ballet training legacy this way:

> Christian Johansson, who conducted the "class of perfection" for the most accomplished dancers of both sexes, was himself the pupil of the Danish ballet master August Bournonville, son of Antoine Bournonville, who in turn was a pupil of Jean Georges Noverre and Auguste Vestris. That is how the direct line of artistic succession from the first sources of the classic ballet art of Noverre, Vestris, Maximilien Gardel and Bournonville was handed down from master to master and was safeguarded and preserved by Petipa and Johansson, who were my contemporaries despite the great difference in our ages.
>
> Carlos Blasis was also represented in the person of Enrico Cecchetti, instructor for the girls' classes and himself the pupil of Giovanni Lepri, a pupil of Blasis. In addition to the old school of Carlo Blasis, Cecchetti also introduced into the Russian ballet the enthusiasm for virtuosity which was characteristic of his own, more recent, style of Italian ballet.
>
> Fokine, *Memoirs*, 24.

18. Shearer, interview by Harris, transcript, 95–96.

19. Quoted in Newman, *Striking a Balance*, 120. Both the de Basil and René Blum companies came into being after the death of Sergei Diaghilev in 1929. "Initially, they drew their personnel from people who had been with Diaghilev or been trained by Russian emigrées." Jackson, Preface, xvi–xvii.

20. Vera Nemchinova was born in Moscow in 1899 and died in New York in 1984. Although she was not a product of the Imperial Theatre Ballet School, Nemchinova was recruited in 1915, at age fifteen, to dance in the corps de ballet of Diaghilev's Ballets Russes. In 1921 she was promoted to ballerina and continued throughout her career to dance with luminaries such as Léonide Massine and Mikhail Mordkin. With another Diaghilev dancer, Anton Dolin, she formed the Nemchinova-Dolin Ballet. She also danced for a time with René Blum's Ballets de Monte Carlo and with the de Basil company. She became a noted teacher in New York City. Pierson, "Nemchinova."

André Eglevsky was born in Moscow in 1917 and died in New York in 1977. Known as an outstanding classical dancer, he was also an exemplary *danseur noble*. He was accepted into the de Basil Ballets Russes de Monte Carlo at age fourteen and furthered his study with Nicolas Legat and Mikhail Fokine. He became a noted teacher and spent many years teaching at George Balanchine's School of American Ballet as well as at his own school in Long Island, New York. Hastings, "Eglevsky."

21. Quoted in Newman, *Striking a Balance,* 120.

22. Craig-Raymond, "Career of Moira Shearer," 3.

23. Quoted in Newman, *Striking a Balance,* 118

24. Quoted in Newman, *Striking a Balance,* 119.

25. Nicholas Sergeyev was born 1876 and graduated from the Imperial Theatre School in 1894. In 1914 he was promoted to first dancer and *régisseur.* Soviet sources have very little that is positive to say about Sergeyev and his relationship to the new ballet of Michel Fokine and the ballet reformers. However, he left Russia in 1918, carrying with him Stepanov notations that he used to restage numerous ballets in the West. These included many of the renowned classics of the late nineteenth century: *The Sleeping Beauty* for the Diaghilev Ballets Russes and for the Sadler's Wells Ballet; *Swan Lake* for Sadler's Wells and for the International Ballet; *Giselle* for the Sadler's Wells and for the Ballet Russe de Monte Carlo, among many others.

26. Quoted in Newman, *Striking a Balance,* 119–20.

27. Kavanaugh, *Secret Muses,* 346.

28. De Valois, *Step by Step,* 16.

29. Ibid., 19.

30. Ibid., 21 (quote). Bronislava Nijinska was the sister of Vaslav Nijinsky and often served as a choreographic assistant to him. But, most important, she was a significant teacher and choreographer in her own right. De Valois studied with Nijinska when the latter was, for a time, choreographing for the Diaghilev Ballets Russes. Nijinska returned to Russia, where she remained during the Revolution and civil war. In 1919 she opened an "experimental" ballet school, the School of Movement, in Kiev. She emigrated to the West in 1921. For more on Nijinska, see Baer, *Bronislava Nijinska.*

31. Ibid., 24 (quote). Olga Preobrajenska was born in 1871 in St. Petersburg and died in 1962 in France. She graduated from the Imperial Theatre School in 1889; she was made soloist there in 1896 and prima ballerina in 1900. She was one of the leading dancers at the turn of the century and took major roles in works of Petipa, Ivanov, the Legats, and Fokine. She herself was the product of training under Cecchetti, Nicolas Legat, Caterina Beretta in Milan, Joseph Hansen in Paris, and Katti Lanner in London. She emigrated in 1922 and danced in major European opera houses and in South America. From 1923 on, she lived in Paris, where she founded her own school. Kulakov, "Preobrajenska."

32. Quoted in Walker, *Ninette de Valois,* 210.

33. Hurok, *S. Hurok Presents,* 290.

34. Of Duncan, Rambert wrote, "When Isadora danced you felt as though she was carried by the music without any effort on her part. I had the feeling that it was as easy as walking, and the grace of it was like a bird's flight. . . . The grace of her movements, and the peaceful happiness of her mood . . . created a complete world of its own—and yet recognisably antique." Rambert, *Quicksilver,* 35. On Diaghilev, Rambert wrote,

> Diaghilev invited me to Berlin to watch a performance of his company with him, and afterwards at supper we discussed what shape my work might take. He listened politely, even sympathetically, to my stupid prejudiced criticism. I said I thought

that the procession in *Cléopâtre* should have corresponded more exactly to the rhythm of the music, which was how Dalcroze would have done it. . . . *L'Après Midi d'une Faune* was also in the programme. Here, the discrepancy between the impressionistic music of Debussy and Nijinsky's absolute austerity of style quite shocked me at the time. *Carnaval,* which came afterwards, enchanted me. I readily accepted Diaghilev's invitation to join the company, to acquaint them with Dalcroze's method, to help Nijinsky in applying it in the production of Stravinsky's *Sacre du Printemps* and to dance in ballets for which I was suitable. Ibid., 54.

35. Bland, "Marie Rambert," 58. "Alexander Bland" is the nom-de-plume of the South African–born dancer and writer Maude Lloyd and her husband, Nigel Gosling, who together wrote about dance until Gosling's death in 1982.

36. Ibid., 61.

37. De Valois, *Come Dance,* 45.

38. Ibid., 47.

39. Franks, *Approach to the Ballet,* 123.

40. De Valois, *Come Dance,* 75.

41. Ibid., 81–82.

42. Walker, *Ninette de Valois,* 104.

43. On Tudor, see Vaughan, *Frederick Ashton,* 120. Daneman writes that according to de Valois, Fonteyn's early talent seemed "average." The future ballerina had other qualities, however, that made her attractive to de Valois. Fonteyn's "judgement was acute, and her way of conducting herself beyond reproach." De Valois was impressed with her ability to "listen." "She knew the people she *shouldn't* listen to. Always very quiet in everything she said. A very balanced person." Daneman, *Margot Fonteyn,* 155.

44. Peter Craig-Raymond reported in *Ballet Today,* "It was during the first crowded year at Covent Garden that Michael Powell, looking for a star for his film *The Red Shoes,* went to the ballet and knew that he had found her. But it took him nearly a year to persuade Moira to accept the part. The film was a phenomenal success, breaking many records, and running for over two years on Broadway. The credit was for the most part, due to Moira Shearer, who became internationally famous and was besieged with film contracts. All these she refused." Craig-Raymond, "Career of Moira Shearer," 19.

45. Quoted in Newman, *Striking a Balance,* 124.

46. Daneman, *Margot Fonteyn,* 202.

47. Craig-Raymond, "Career of Moira Shearer," 19. In fact, she did go on to make other films: another Powell-Pressburger collaboration, *The Tales of Hoffman* (1950); *The Story of Three Loves* (directed by Gottfried Reinhardt, 1952); *The Man Who Loved Redheads* (directed by Harold French, 1954); *Peeping Tom* (directed by Michael Powell, 1960); and *Black Tights* (directed by Terence Young, 1960).

48. Ibid.

49. On the discomfort Shearer endured in making *The Red Shoes,* see Turner, "'The Red Shoes,'" 105.

50. Daneman, *Margot Fonteyn,* 220–21.

51. Photo from unidentified magazine, clippings file, MGZR Shearer, Moira, New York Public Library–Dance Division.

52. Daneman, *Margot Fonteyn,* 202–3.

53. Quoted, ibid., 229.

54. The *pas de trois* "Florestan and His Two Sisters" was an addition by Ashton, choreographed for the 1946 production at Covent Garden. It was danced by Moira Shearer, Gerd Larsen, and Michael Somes, replacing the Jewel Fairies' *pas de quatre* in act 3. Vaughan, *Frederick Ashton*, 202–3.

55. Quoted in Daneman, *Margot Fonteyn*, 236.

56. Shearer, interview by Harris, transcript, 20.

57. Quoted in Daneman, *Margot Fonteyn*, 236–37.

58. Elvin, interview by Dale Harris, August 9–11, 1978, transcript, 22–23, New York Public Library, Performing Arts Center.

59. Ibid., 115–16.

60. Macaulay, *Margot Fonteyn*, 27.

61. Daneman, *Margot Fonteyn*, 237.

62. Fonteyn, *Autobiography*, 107.

63. Quoted in Daneman, *Margot Fonteyn*, 263.

64. Quoted in Newman, *Striking a Balance*, 122.

65. Regarding the first tour to New York, for instance, one former company member, Leslie Edwards, writes, "The success of Margot Fonteyn during this season has been well documented, but it must not be forgotten that the company included a number of really notable dancers. . . . Each ballerina gained her own following with an individual interpretation of the great classical rôles: Pamela May, Beryl Grey, Violetta Elvin, Nadia Nerina—and Moira Shearer, who had a special rapport with the American audiences, not surprisingly, considering her success on the screen." Edwards, *In Good Company*, 133.

66. Elvin, interview by Harris, transcript, 22–23.

67. Shearer, interview by Harris, transcript, 20. Olga Spessivtseva was born in Rostov in 1895 and died in 1991 in New York. After studying at the Imperial Theatre School, she joined the Maryinsky Ballet Company in 1913. In 1916 she was made a soloist and that year danced for the first time with Sergei Diaghilev's Ballets Russes. Noted as a supreme classicist, she was appreciated for her air of fragility and melancholy and was particularly known for her role in *Giselle*. A remarkably successful dancer, she received an early promotion to prima ballerina in 1920. She left Russia permanently in 1924 and left Europe at the beginning of World War II to settle in New York, where she served as an advisor to Ballet Theatre. Troubled with mental illness, Spessivtseva was hospitalized from 1942 to 1963. After her release she lived in New York State. Dorvane, "Olga Spessivtseva."

68. Shearer's very evident success when the company performed in New York's cavernous Metropolitan Opera House belies such claims.

69. Quoted in Newman, *Striking a Balance*, 123.

70. Ibid., 130.

71. Haskell, "Outstanding Events of the Year," 11.

72. Williamson, *Ballet Renaissance*, 53–54.

73. Clarke, *Sadler's Wells Ballet*, 204.

74. Vaughan, *Frederick Ashton*, 231.

75. Clarke, *Sadler's Wells Ballet*, 230–32.

76. Macaulay, *Margot Fonteyn*, 44.

77. Hurok, S. *Hurok Presents,* 240.

78. De Valois, *Come Dance,* 180.

79. In a 1969 postcript to the review, first published in 1949, Haggin added that he had reconsidered this first impression. He wrote that he found the ballet "feeble, inane and boring." Haggin, *Ballet Chronicle,* 16.

80. Ibid.

81. Vaughan, *Frederick Ashton,* 208–9.

82. Clarke, *Sadler's Wells Ballet,* 207.

83. Quoted in Newman, *Striking a Balance,* 134.

84. Ibid., 125.

85. Ibid., 126–27.

86. Ibid., 127.

87. Ibid. Of this incident, Alistair Macauley writes, "Shearer reserves all her criticism for de Valois here; still, one must wonder just how free Fonteyn can have been from complicity in this arrangement." Macauley, *Margot Fonteyn,* 50.

88. Quoted in Newman, *Striking a Balance,* 127.

89. Shearer, interview by Harris, transcript, 33.

90. Haskell, *Ballet Annual 1949,* 37.

91. Clarke, *Sadler's Wells Ballet,* 249.

92. Monahan, *Fonteyn,* 36.

93. Shearer later wrote a book about Balanchine entitled *Balletmaster: A Dancer's View of George Balanchine* (1986).

94. Shearer, interview by Harris, transcript, 108.

95. Ibid., 109.

96. Ibid.

97. Ibid., 113.

98. Ibid, 114.

99. Ibid., 87.

CHAPTER 5: CATHERINE KERR

1. Cunningham, *Changes,* n.p.

2. Catherine Kerr, interview by author, New York, N.Y., July 27, 1998.

3. Ibid.

4. Ibid.

5. Ibid. I use the term "postmodern" in an effort to distinguish Laura Dean's generation of artists from that of Merce Cunningham and John Cage. Cunningham and Cage, though often "wildly" experimental, frequently served as mentors and teachers to the postmoderns and minimalists. Sally Banes describes Dean as one of the many dancemakers "actively involved in the creation of the post-modern aesthetic." Like Lucinda Childs and Kenneth King, Laura Dean, in the 1970s, says Banes, operated as "a geometer," "tracing distinct designs in a well-controlled space." Banes, "Introduction: Sources of Post-Modern Dance," in *Terpsichore in Sneakers,* 18–19.

6. Kerr, interview by author, July 27, 1998.

7. Vaughan, *Merce Cunningham,* 186. Cunningham described the origin of the Events: In 1964 the company was invited to perform at the Twentieth Century Museum in

Vienna. The space was not amenable to the performance of full repertory works. "The audience had no place to go at the intermissions, there was no curtain, no wings, no lights, no place to put scenery. So I thought we'd just do the pieces that we had with us, one on top of another, for an hour and a half." The Events were "parts of pieces, sometimes we doubled, we had two dances going on at the same time," and were performed without intermission and without conventional proscenium stage. Quoted in Lesschaeve, *Dancer and the Dance*, 175.

8. Vaughan, *Merce Cunningham*, 189, 190.

9. Banes writes, "The Early Sixties avant-garde artists did not aim passively to reflect the society they lived in; they tried to change it by producing a new culture." Banes, *Greenwich Village 1963*, 10.

10. For comprehensive biographical and choreographic information, see Vaughan, *Merce Cunningham*.

11. According to one analysis, "The central thesis sustaining [Graham's] work was that the function of dance was communication—that it must speak to the mind and emotions and body of the spectator in terms transcending words." Reynolds and McCormick, *No Fixed Points*, 146.

12. The Judson Dance Theater, named for the Judson Church in New York's Greenwich Village, was launched on July 6, 1962. The group came together as students of the musician Robert Dunn, himself a student of John Cage. The first concert that resulted from Dunn's "stimulating and unorthodox composition class" was a historic three-and-a-half-hour performance featuring twenty-one works by fourteen choreographers, including a film by Elaine Summers. Deborah Jowitt says the concert "excited" some spectators and "horrified others." Many felt threatened. As Jowitt says, "Virtuosity—and with it almost anything that looked like 'dance technique'—was out. So were role-playing and acting and glamour." Jowitt, *Time and the Dancing Image*, 309.

13. David Vaughan believes that what aligned Cage and Cunningham with Duchamp was their shared avoidance of self-reflexive art. He quotes Calvin Tomkins, who wrote that the works of abstract expressionist artists such as Jackson Pollock took as their theme "the heroically suffering artist." Instead, says Vaughan, Cage and Cunningham, like Duchamp, investigated the possibilities of the forms themselves. Duchamp's readymades and the Cage-Cunningham chance operations allowed these artists to "erase the distinction between art and life," and got them away from a focus on the artistic ego. Vaughan, "'Then I Thought About Marcel,'" 67.

14. Tomkins, *Bride and the Bachelors*, 73.

15. Although Cunningham is not interested in art that imposes an artificial sense of meaning, he does not deny "passion," or "emotion" in movement: "you do not separate the human being from the actions he does, or the actions which surround him, but you can see what it is like to break these actions up in different ways, to allow the passion, and it is passion, to appear for each person in his own way." Cunningham, *Changes*, n.p.

16. See Novack, *Sharing the Dance*, for an examination of the origins of Contact Improvisation, a movement form that developed in the 1960s and was partly stimulated by interest in Asian martial arts and Eastern philosophy.

17. Tomkins, *Bride and the Bachelors*, 73.

18. Banes, "Dancing in the Museum," 14. Banes continues, "Cunningham's students

and younger colleagues at the Judson Dance Theater, a choreographic collective that presented experimental dance by artists and musicians as well as trained dancers, challenged traditional uses of space even further by rejecting conventional stage altogether. They danced purely secular dances in church sanctuaries, and also in roller-skating rinks, in lofts, and in art museums, including (in 1966) the Walker Art Center—to the consternation of critics, who found their rejection of theatrical space impertinent." Ibid.

19. Cunningham, "Four Events."

20. Tomkins, "On Collaboration," 45.

21. Cunningham, "Four Events." Also significant for Cunningham are his experiments with video and film work that began in the 1970s. While the camera has its limits, he said, "It also can show dance in a way not always possible on the stage: that is, the use of detail which in the broader context of theatre does not appear." Since the 1990s Cunningham has used the "Life-Forms" computer program. The computer allows him to "make up movements, put them in the memory [and] eventually have a phrase of movement. This can be examined from any angle, including overhead." The figure on the computer can "produce shapes and transitions that are not available on humans, but as happened first with the rhythmic structure, then with the use of chance operations, followed by the use of the camera on film and video and now with the dance computer, I am aware once more of new possibilities with which to work." As Cunningham summed up, "My work has always been in process. Finishing a dance has left me with the idea, often slim in the beginning, for the next one. In that way, I do not think of each dance as an object, rather a short stop on the way." Ibid..

22. Copeland, *Merce Cunningham*, 79–80.

23. Flett, "Shaping Up to Merce."

24. Cunningham, quoted in Tomkins, "On Collaboration," 47.

25. Lise Friedman danced in Cunningham's company from 1977 to 1984 and was often paired with Kerr. Friedman's lush, adagio movement quality offset Kerr's powerful physicality. The two were complementary; when they shared a role, their individual movement qualities revealed the richness inherent in Cunningham's choreography.

26. Lise Friedman, interview by author, New York, N.Y., October 4, 2001.

27. Quoted in Kuhn, "Cunningham in Conversation," 23.

28. Friedman, interview by author.

29. Vaughan, "Retrospect and Prospect," 125.

30. Vaughan, *Merce Cunningham*, 193.

31. Reed, "Over Your Head,." The quotation in the next paragraph is from the same source.

32. Kitty Cunningham, "Merce Cunningham and Dance Company," 44.

33. Macaulay, "Merce Cunningham," 734.

34. Willinger, *Ballet News*.

35. Lesschaeve, *Dancer and the Dance*, 156.

36. Vaughan, *Merce Cunningham*, 213.

37. Greskovic, "Merce Cunningham as Sculptor," 95.

38. Kerr, interview by author, New York, N.Y., October 7, 2001.

39. Ibid.

40. *Doubles* was commissioned by the American Dance Festival as part of its fiftieth-anniversary celebration; it was first performed in 1984.

41. Friedman, interview by author.

42. Julie Kavanaugh, review, *Spectator,* June 1, 1985; Jennifer Dunning, review, *New York Times,* August 9, 1984.

43. Tobias, "Love at First Sight," 72. Robert Swinston has danced in the Merce Cunningham Dance Company (hereafter, MCDC) since 1980. Today he also serves as assistant to the choreographer.

44. Kriegsman, "Dance in Performance."

45. Aloff, "Merce Cunningham Dance Company," 603.

46. Kerr, interview by author, October 7, 2001.

47. Ibid.

48. On the video this partner is Kevin Schroder, who danced with MCDC during 1985–86.

49. Macaulay, "Merce Experience," 1051. Alan Good danced with MCDC from 1978 to 1989.

50. Kerr, interview by author, July 27, 1998.

51. Ibid.

52. Friedman, interview by author.

53. Kerr, interview by author, October 7, 2001. Viola Farber danced with MCDC from 1953 to 1965 and returned as a guest artist in January 1970 to perform in a revival of Cunningham's *Crises* (1960).

54. Friedman, interview by author. Joseph Lennon danced with MCDC from 1978 to 1984.

55. Ibid.

56. Ibid.

57. Kerr, interview by author, October 7, 2001.

58. Jacobs, "Cunningham and Kandinsky," 23.

59. Lewis, "Merce Cunningham Company."

60. Kerr, interview by author, October 7, 2001.

61. Lewis, "Merce Cunningham Company" ("supertechnicians"); Cunningham quoted in Lesschaeve, *Dancer and the Dance,* 68 ("movement operates").

62. Foster, *Reading Dancing,* 48 (quote).

EPILOGUE

1. Carter, "Destabilising the Discipline," in *Rethinking Dance History,* 16.

2. For an account of the deliberate decision to create a sense of tradition and history in British ballet, see Genné, "Creating a Canon."

BIBLIOGRAPHY

Aloff, Mindy. "Merce Cunningham Dance Company." *Nation,* May 18, 1985, 603–4.

Andrieux, Maurice. *Daily Life in Venice in the Time of Casanova.* Translated by Mary Fitton. New York: Praeger, 1972.

Arkin, Lisa, and Marian Smith, "National Dance in the Romantic Ballet." In Garafola, *Rethinking the Sylph,* 11–68.

Baer, Nancy Van Norman. *Bronislava Nijinska: A Dancer's Legacy.* San Francisco: Fine Arts Museum of San Francisco, 1986.

Banes, Sally. "Dancing in the Museum: The Impure Art." In *Art Performs Life: Merce Cunningham/Meredith Monk/Bill T. Jones,* 10–15. New York: Distributed Art Publishers, 1998.

———. *Dancing Women: Female Bodies on Stage.* New York: Routledge, 1998.

———. *Greenwich Village 1963: Avant-Garde Performance and the Effervescent Body.* Durham: Duke University Press, 1993.

———. *Terpsichore in Sneakers: Post-Modern Dance.* Hanover, N.H.: Wesleyan University Press, 1987.

Baudelaire, Charles. *The Painter of Modern Life and Other Essays.* Translated by Jonathan Mayne. London: Phaidon, 1995.

Baur-Heinhold, Margarete. *The Baroque Theatre: A Cultural History of the Seventeenth and Eighteenth Centuries.* New York: McGraw-Hill, 1967.

Beaumont, Cyril W. *The Ballet Called Giselle.* 1945. Reprint, Brooklyn: Dance Horizons, 1969.

———. *The Complete Book of Ballets.* New York: Grosset and Dunlap, 1938.

Benois, Alexandre. *Memoirs.* Translated by Moura Budberg. London: Chatto and Windus, 1960.

Bentley, Toni. *Winter Season: A Dancer's Journal.* New York: Random House, 1982.

Binney, Edwin. *Glories of the Romantic Ballet.* London: Dance Books, 1985.

Bland, Alexander. "Marie Rambert." In Haskell, *The Ballet Annual,* vol. 9, 58–63.

Bournonville, August. *Letters on Dance and Choreography.* Translated by Knud Arne Jürgensen. London: Dance Books, 1999.

———. *A New Year's Gift for Dance Lovers or A View of the Dance as Fine Art and Pleasant Pastime.* Translated by Inge Biller Kelly. London: Royal Academy of Dancing, 1977.

Bruce, H. J. *Thirty Dozen Moons.* London: Constable, 1949.

Buckle, Richard. *Diaghilev.* New York: Atheneum, 1979.

———. *In the Wake of Diaghilev.* New York: Holt, Rinehart, and Winston, 1982.

———. *Nijinsky.* New York: Simon and Schuster, 1971.

Burnim, Kalman A., and Philip H. Highfill Jr. *John Bell, Patron of British Theatrical Portraiture: A Catalog of the Theatrical Portraits in his Editions of Bell's Shakespeare and Bell's British Theatre.* Carbondale: Southern Illinois University Press, 1998.

Carter, Alexandra, ed. *Rethinking Dance History: A Reader.* New York: Routledge, 2004.

Castil-Blaze. *L'Académie impériale de musique.* Paris, 1855.

Chapman, John V. "Auguste Vestris and the Expansion of Technique." *Dance Research Journal* 19, no. 1 (Summer 1987): 11–18.

———. "Forgotten Giant: Pierre Gardel." *Dance Research* 5, no. 1 (Spring 1987): 3–20.

———. "Jules Janin: Romantic Critic." In Garafola, *Rethinking the Sylph,* 197–241.

Chazin-Bennahum, Judith. *Dance in the Shadow of the Guillotine.* Carbondale: Southern Illinois University Press, 1988.

Christie, Ian. *Arrows of Desire: The Films of Michael Powell and Emeric Pressburger.* London: Waterstone, 1985.

Clarke, Mary. *The Sadler's Wells Ballet: A History and an Appreciation.* London: Adam and Charles Black, 1955.

———. *Six Great Dancers.* London: Hamish Hamilton, 1957.

Cohen, Sarah R. *Art, Dance, and the Body in French Culture of the Ancien Régime.* New York: Cambridge University Press, 2000.

Cohen, Selma Jeanne, ed. *International Encyclopedia of Dance.* 6 vols. New York: Oxford University Press, 1998.

Copeland, Roger. *Merce Cunningham: The Modernizing of Modern Dance.* New York: Routledge, 2004.

Craig-Raymond, Peter. "The Career of Moira Shearer." *Ballet Today,* December 1954, 3, 19, 21.

Cranston, Maurice. *The Romantic Movement.* Cambridge: Blackwell, 1994.

Cunningham, Kitty. "Merce Cunningham and Dance Company around New York." *Dance and Dancers,* August 1974, 43–44.

Cunningham, Merce. *Changes: Notes on Choreography.* New York: Something Else Press, 1968.

———. "Four Events That Have Led to Large Discoveries." In Vaughan, *Merce Cunningham,* 276.

Dalla Valle, Tino. "La fama vien danzando." *Il Resto del Carlino* (Bologna), December 16, 1976.

Daneman, Meredith. *Margot Fonteyn: A Life.* New York: Viking, 2004.

Davenport, Millia. *The Book of Costume.* Vol. 1. New York: Crown, 1948.

Davis, Natalie Zemon. *Women on the Margins: Three Seventeenth-Century Lives.* Cambridge, Mass.: Harvard University Press, 1995.

De Valois, Ninette. *Come Dance with Me: A Memoir, 1898–1956.* Cleveland: World, 1957.

———. *Step by Step: The Formation of an Establishment.* London: W. H. Allen, 1977.

Dorvane, Jeannine. "Spessivtseva, Olga." In Cohen, *International Encyclopedia of Dance.*

Drummond, John. *Speaking of Diaghilev.* London: Faber and Faber, 1998.

Dunning, Jennifer. "In 'Giselle,' the Acting Informs the Dance." *New York Times,* May 21, 2001.

Duplain. "Guimard, ou L'Art de la danse-pantomime." 1783. Bibliothèque de l'Opéra, Paris.

Edwards, Leslie, with Graham Bowles. *In Good Company: Sixty Years with the Royal Ballet.* Hampshire, Eng.: Dance Books, 2003.

Eglevsky, André, and John Gregory. *Heritage of a Ballet Master: Nicholas Legat.* New York: Dance Horizons, 1977.

Einberg, Elizabeth. *Gainsborough's Giovanna Baccelli.* London: Tate Gallery, 1976.

Elvin, Violetta. Interview by Dale Harris, August 1978. Transcript. New York Public Library, Performing Arts Division.

Fairfax, Edmund. *The Styles of Eighteen-Century Ballet.* Lanham, Md.: Scarecrow Press, 2003.

Farge, Arlette. *Fragile Lives: Violence, Power, and Solidarity in Eighteenth-Century Paris.* Translated by Carol Shelton. Cambridge Mass.: Harvard University Press, 1993.

Figes, Orlando. *Natasha's Dance: A Cultural History of Russia.* Henry Holt, 2002.

Flett, Una. "Shaping Up to Merce." *Scotsman,* September 7, 1979.

Fokine, Michel. *Fokine: Memoirs of a Ballet Master.* Translated by Vitale Fokine. London: Constable, 1961.

Fonteyn, Margot. *Autobiography.* New York: Knopf, 1976.

Foreman, Amanda. *Georgiana Duchess of Devonshire.* London: Harper Collins, 1999.

Foster, Susan. *Reading Dancing: Bodies and Subjects in Contemporary American Dance.* Berkeley: University of California Press, 1986.

Franks, A. H. *Approach to the Ballet.* London: Sir Isaac Pitman and Sons, 1948.

Gaddis, John Lewis. *The Landscape of History: How Historians Map the Past.* New York: Oxford University Press, 2002.

Gallini, Giovanni-Andrea. *A Treatise on the Art of Dancing.* 1762. New York: Broude, 1967.

Garafola, Lynn. *Diaghilev's Ballets Russes.* 1989. New York: Da Capo, 1998.

———. "Reconfiguring the Sexes." In *The Ballets Russes and Its World,* edited by Lynn Garafola and Nancy Van Norman Baer, 245–68. New Haven: Yale University Press, 1999.

———, ed. *Rethinking the Sylph: New Perspectives on the Romantic Ballet.* Hanover, N.H.: Wesleyan University Press, 1997.

———. "The Travesty Dancer in Nineteenth-Century Ballet." *Dance Research Journal* 17, no. 2, and 18, no. 1 (1985–86): 35–40.

Gautier, Théophile. *Gautier on Dance*. Edited by Ivor Guest. London: Dance Books, 1986.

———. *Histoire de l'art dramatique en France depuis vingt-cinq ans.* Vol. 3. Leipzig: Edition Hetzel, 1859.

———. *Mademoiselle de Maupin*. Translated by Joanna Richardson. New York: Penguin, 1981.

Genné, Beth. "Creating a Canon, Creating the 'Classics' in Twentieth-Century British Ballet." *Dance Research* 18, no. 2 (Winter 2000): 132–62.

Gerkin, Eva. "Chambermaids for Hire." *Opera News*, February 25, 1961, 21.

Greskovic, Robert. "Merce Cunningham as Sculptor." *Ballet Review* (Winter 1984): 88–95.

Grigoriev, S. L. *The Diaghilev Ballet, 1909–1929*. Translated by Vera Bowen. Baltimore: Penguin, 1960.

Guest, Ivor. *The Ballet of the Enlightenment: The Establishment of the Ballet d'Action in France, 1770–1793*. London: Dance Books, 1996.

———. *Ballet of the Second Empire*. London: Pitman, 1974.

———. *A Gallery of Romantic Ballet: A Catalogue of the Collection of Dance Prints at the Mercury Theatre*. London: New Mercury, 1965.

———. "The Italian Lady of Knole." In *The Ballet Annual: A Record and Year Book of the Ballet*, edited by Arnold Haskell, vol. 11, 78–85. London: Adam and Charles Black, 1957.

———. *Jules Perrot: Master of the Romantic Ballet*. New York: Dance Horizons, 1984.

———. *The Romantic Ballet in Paris*. Middletown, Conn.: Wesleyan University Press, 1966.

———. *Victorian Ballet Girl: The Tragic Story of Clara Webster*. London: Adam and Charles Black, 1957.

Haggin, B. H. *Ballet Chronicle*. New York: Horizon, 1970.

Hallet, Mark. "Reynolds, Celebrity and the Exhibition Space." In *Joshua Reynolds: The Creation of Celebrity*, edited by Martin Postle, 35–47. London: Tate Publishing, 2005.

Hammond, Sandra Noll. "Clues to Ballet's Technical History from the Early Nineteenth Century Ballet Lesson." *Dance Research* 3, no. 1 (Autumn 1984): 53–66.

———. "Searching for the Sylph: Documentation of Early Developments in Pointe Technique." *Dance Research Journal* 19, no. 2 (Winter 1987–88): 27–31.

Haskell, Arnold, ed. *The Ballet Annual: A Record and Year Book of the Ballet*. Vol. 1. London: Adam and Charles Black, 1949.

———. *The Ballet Annual: A Record and Year Book of the Ballet*. Vol. 9. London: Adam and Charles Black, 1955.

———. *Balletomania Then and Now*. New York: Knopf, 1977.

———. "Outstanding Events of the Year: Sadler's Wells at Covent Garden." In *Ballet Decade*, edited by Arnold Haskell, 10–12. New York: Macmillan, 1946.

Haskell, Arnold, and Walter Nouvel. *Diaghileff: His Artistic and Private Life*. New York: Simon and Schuster, 1935.

Hastings, Baird. "Eglevsky, André." In Cohen, *International Encyclopedia of Dance*.

Hering, Doris. "Dancing the Classics, American Ballet Theatre." *Dance Magazine*, April 1976.

Highfill, Philip H., Kalman A. Burnim, and Edward A. Langhans. *A Biographical Dictionary of Actors, Actresses, Musicians, Dancers, Managers and Other Stage Personnel in London, 1660–1800.* Carbondale: Southern Illinois University Press, 1973–93.

Higonnet, Anne. "Representations of Women." In *Emerging Feminism from Revolution to World War,* edited by Genevieve Fraisse and Michelle Perrot. Vol. 4 of *History of Women in the West.* Cambridge, Mass.: Belknap Press, 1993.

Huckenpahler, Victoria, ed. "Confessions of an Opera Director: Chapters from the Mémoires of Dr. Louis Véron, Part One." *Dance Chronicle* 7, no. 1 (1984): 50–106.

———. "Confessions of an Opera Director: Chapters from the Mémoires of Dr. Louis Véron, Part Three." *Dance Chronicle* 7, no. 3 (1984–85): 345–70.

Hurok, Sol. *S. Hurok Presents: A Memoir of the Dance World.* New York: Hermitage House, 1953.

Jackson, George. Preface. *The One and Only: The Ballet Russe de Monte Carlo,* by Jack Anderson. London: Dance Books, 1981.

Jacobs, Laura A. "Cunningham and Kandinsky." *New Leader,* April 8, 1985, 22–23.

Jowitt, Deborah. *Time and the Dancing Image.* Berkeley: University of California Press, 1988.

Jürgensen, Knud Arne. *The Bournonville Tradition: The First Fifty Years, 1829–1879.* Vol. 1. London: Dance Books, 1997.

Kahane, Martine. *Le foyer de la danse.* Paris: Musée d'Orsay, 1988.

Karsavina, Tamara. *Ballet Technique: A Series of Practical Essays.* London: Adam and Charles Black, 1956.

———. *Theatre Street.* 1931. New York: Dutton, 1961.

———. "Why 'Ballet Russe' Could Not Survive Diaghileff." In Haskell, *The Ballet Annual,* vol. 9, 50–57.

Kavanaugh, Julie. *Secret Muses: The Life of Frederick Ashton.* New York: Pantheon, 1996.

Kisselgoff, Anna. "A Dance of Remorse and Regeneration." *New York Times,* July 20, 2000.

Koritz, Amy. *Gendering Bodies/Performing Art: Dance and Literature in Early Twentieth-Century British Culture.* Ann Arbor: University of Michigan Press, 1995.

Kostelanetz, Richard, ed. *Merce Cunningham: Dancing in Space and Time.* Pennington, N.J.: A Cappella Books, 1992.

Kriegsman, Alan M. "Dance in Performance: The Master and His Moves." *Washington Post,* March 30, 1985.

Kschssinska, Mathilde. *Dancing in Petersburg: The Memoirs of Kschessinska.* Translated by Arnold Haskell. London: Victor Gollancz, 1960.

Kuhn, Laura. "Merce Cunningham in Conversation with Laura Kuhn." In *Art Performs Life: Merce Cunningham/Meredith Monk/Bill T. Jones,* edited by Laura Kuhn, 22–65. New York: Distributed Art Publishers, 1998.

Kulakov, Valery. "Preobrajenska, Olga." In Cohen, *International Encyclopedia of Dance.*

Kyasht, Lydia. *Romantic Recollections.* New York: Da Capo, 1978.

Lesschaeve, Jacqueline. *The Dancer and the Dance: Merce Cunningham in Conversation with Jacqueline Lesschaeve.* New York: Marion Boyars, 1985.

Lewis, Maggie. "Merce Cunningham Company: The Supertechnicians of Dance." *Christian Science Monitor,* November 21, 1985.

Lieven, Peter. *The Birth of the Ballets-Russes*. New York: Dover, 1973.

Lincoln, W. Bruce. *The Romanovs: Autocrats of All the Russias*. New York: Doubleday, 1981.

———. *Sunlight at Midnight: St. Petersburg and the Rise of Modern Russia*. New York: Basic Books, 2000.

Lindsay, Jack. *Thomas Gainsborough: His Life and Art*. London: Granada, 1981.

Lowe, Alfonso. *La Serenissima: The Last Flowering of the Venetian Republic*. London: Cassell, 1974.

Lumley, Benjamin. *Reminiscences of the Opera*. London: Hurst and Plackett, 1864.

Lynham, Deryck. *The Chevalier Noverre: Father of Modern Ballet*. London: Sylvan Press, 1950.

Macaulay, Alistair. *Margot Fonteyn*. Gloucestershire, Eng.: Sutton, 1998.

———. "Merce Cunningham, First Impressions." *Dancing Times*, August 1980, 734–35.

———. "The Merce Experience." *Dancing Times*, September 1987, 1050–52.

Magri, Gennaro. *Theoretical and Practical Treatise on Dancing*. Naples, 1799. Translated by Mary Skeaping. London: Dance Books, 1988.

Maurice, Charles. *Histoire anecdotique de théatre de la littérature et de diverse impressions contemporaines tirée du Coffre d'un journaliste avec sa vie à tort et à travers Charles Maurice*. Paris: Henri Plon, 1856.

McDonald, Nesta. *Diaghilev Observed by Critics in England and the United States, 1911–1929*. New York: Dance Horizons, 1975.

McMillan, James F. *France and Women, 1789–1914: Gender, Society and Politics*. New York: Routledge, 1998.

Migel, Parmenia. *The Ballerinas*. New York: Macmillan, 1972.

Monahan, James. *Fonteyn: A Study of the Ballerina in Her Setting*. London: Adam and Charles Black, 1957.

Morrison, Toni. "The Site of Memory." In *Out There: Marginalization and Contemporary Cultures*, edited by Russell Ferguson, Martha Gever, Trinh T. Minh-ha, and Cornel West, 299–305. Cambridge, Mass.: MIT Press, 1990.

Newman, Barbara. *Striking a Balance: Dancers Talk about Dancing*. New York: Limelight Editions, 1992.

Novack, Cynthia J. *Sharing the Dance: Contact Improvisation and American Culture*. Madison: University of Wisconsin Press, 1990.

Noverre, Jean-Georges. *Letters on Dancing and Ballets*. St. Petersburg, 1803. Translated and edited by C. W. Beaumont. London: C. W. Beaumont, 1951.

Perrot, Michelle, ed. *From the Fires of Revolution to the Great War*. Translated by Arthur Godhammer. History of Private Life 4. Cambridge, Mass.: Harvard University Press, 1990.

Pierson, Rosalind. "Nemchinova, Vera." In Cohen, *International Dictionary of Ballet*.

Postle, Martin. "'The Modern Apelles': Joshua Reynolds and the Creation of Celebrity." In *Joshua Reynolds: The Creation of Celebrity*, edited by Martin Postle, 17–33. London: Tate Publishing, 2005.

Price, Curtis, Judith Milhous, and Robert D. Hume. *Italian Opera in Late Eighteenth Century London*. Vol. 1: *The King's Theatre, Haymarket, 1778–1791*. Oxford: Clarendon Press. 1995.

Prod'homme, J.-G. *L'Opéra (1669–1925)*. Paris, n.d.

Rambert, Marie. *Quicksilver: An Autobiography*. London: Macmillan, 1972.

Reed, Jim. "Over Your Head, Like the Sun." *Woodstock Times*, June 19, 1980.

Reynolds, Nancy, and Malcolm McCormick. *No Fixed Points: Dance in the Twentieth Century*. New Haven: Yale University Press, 2003.

Robin-Challan, Louise. "Social Conditions of Ballet Dancers at the Paris Opera in the 19th Century." *Choreography and Dance* 2, no. 1 (1992): 17–28.

Rosenthal, Michael, and Martin Myrone, eds. *Gainsborough*. London: Tate Publishing, 2002.

Roslavleva, Natalia. *Era of the Russian Ballet, 1770–1965*. New York: Dutton, 1966.

Royer, Alphonse. *Histoire de l'Opéra*. Paris, 1875.

Sackville-West, Robert. *Knole, Kent*. London: National Trust Enterprises, 1983.

Sackville-West, Vita. *Knole and the Sackvilles*. London: William Heinemann, 1923.

Sand, George. *Indiana*. Edited by Marilyn Yalom. New York: Penguin Books, 1993.

Scholl, Tim. *From Petipa to Balanchine: Classical Revival and the Modernization of Ballet*. New York: Routledge, 1994.

Second, Albéric. *Les petits mystères de l'Opéra*. Paris: G. Kugelmann, 1844.

Shearer, Moira. Interview by Dale Harris. August 1976, August 1978. Transcript. New York Public Library, Performing Arts Division.

Simonton, Deborah. *A History of European Women's Work, 1700 to the Present*. New York: Routledge, 1998.

Smith, Marian. *Ballet and Opera in the Age of Giselle*. Princeton: Princeton University Press, 2000.

Thackeray, William Makepeace. *The Paris Sketch Book of Mr. M. A. Titmarsh; The Irish Sketch Book, And Notes of a Journey from Cornhill to Grand Cairo*. New York: Belford, Clarke, and Co., n.d.

Tobias, Tobi. "Love at First Sight." *New York Magazine*, March 25, 1985.

Tomkins, Calvin. *The Bride and the Bachelors: Five Masters of the Avant-Garde*. 1965. New York: Penguin, 1977.

———. "On Collaboration" (1974). In Kostelanetz, *Merce Cunningham*, 44–47.

Turner, George. "'The Red Shoes': A Ballet for Camera." *American Cinematographer: The International Journal of Film and Digital Production Techniques* 79, no. 2 (February 1998): 102–8.

Vaughan, David. *Frederick Ashton and His Ballets*. New York: Knopf, 1977.

———. *Merce Cunningham: Fifty Years*. New York: Aperture, 1997.

———. "Retrospect and Prospect." 1979. In Kostelanetz, *Merce Cunningham*, 124–31.

———. "'Then I Thought About Marcel . . .' Merce Cunningham's *Walkaround Time*." 1982. In Kostelanetz, *Merce Cunningham*, 66–70.

Walker, Kathrine Sorley. *Ninette de Valois: Idealist without Illusions*. London: Hamish Hamilton, 1987.

Walpole, Horace. *The Yale Editions of Horace Walpole's Correspondence*. 48 vols. Edited by W. S. Lewis et al. New Haven: Yale University Press, 1937–83.

Williamson, Audrey. *Ballet Renaissance*. London: Golden Balley Press, 1948.

Willinger, Edward. Review of *Coast Zone*. *Ballet News*, July 1983, 33–34.

Winter, Marian Hannah. *The Pre-Romantic Ballet*. London: Pitman, 1974.

———. *The Theatre of Marvels*. New York: Benjamin Blom, 1964.

INDEX

KAREN ELIOT is a former member of the
Merce Cunningham Dance Company and
a lifelong dancer. She is a professor of dance
at the Ohio State University, where she
teaches modern and ballet techniques and
dance history.

THE UNIVERSITY OF ILLINOIS PRESS
IS A FOUNDING MEMBER OF THE
ASSOCIATION OF AMERICAN UNIVERSITY PRESSES.

COMPOSED IN 10/13 ADOBE CASLON PRO
WITH FUTURA AND SASSAFRAS DISPLAY
BY JIM PROEFROCK
AT THE UNIVERSITY OF ILLINOIS PRESS
DESIGNED BY COPENHAVER CUMPSTON
MANUFACTURED BY THOMSON-SHORE, INC.

UNIVERSITY OF ILLINOIS PRESS
1325 SOUTH OAK STREET
CHAMPAIGN, IL 61820–6903
WWW.PRESS.UILLINOIS.EDU